Technologies of Pr[...]
Second Edition

Technologies of Procreation brings a fresh approach to the analysis of the social and cultural implications of assisted conception technologies. It explores how these techniques create the potential for a redefinition of relationships, because it is now possible to create life on behalf of another person.

In this Second Edition, the authors have added new sections to each chapter which contain significant material developing upon the original argument. By drawing on data and ideas from ethnographic studies, household interviews, and debates in Parliament and among clinicians, the authors present an innovative approach to the transformations of parenthood, procreation and kinship in the context of new reproductive technologies. *Technologies of Procreation* will be of interest to a wide range of readers in anthropology, sociology, medical ethics and health research.

Jeanette Edwards is in the Department of Sociology and Anthropology at Keele University; **Sarah Franklin** is in the Department of Sociology at Lancaster University; **Eric Hirsch** is in the Department of Human Sciences at Brunel University; **Frances Price** is in the Faculty of Social and Political Sciences at Cambridge University; and **Marilyn Strathern** is in the Department of Social Anthropology at Cambridge University.

Technologies of Procreation

Kinship in the age of assisted conception

Second Edition

Jeanette Edwards, Sarah Franklin, Eric Hirsch, Frances Price, Marilyn Strathern

Routledge

London and New York

First published 1993
by Manchester University Press
Oxford Road, Manchester M13 9PL and
Room 400, 175 Fifth Avenue, New York, NY 10010, USA

Second Edition published 1999
by Routledge
11 New Fetter Lane, London EC4P 4EE

Simultaneously published in the USA and Canada
by Routledge
29 West 35th Street, New York, NY 10001, USA

© 1999 Jeanette Edwards, Sarah Franklin, Eric Hirsch, Frances Price
and Marilyn Strathern

Typeset in Galliard by RefineCatch Limited, Bungay, Suffolk
Printed and bound in Great Britain by
Redwood Books, Trowbridge, Wiltshire

British Library Cataloguing in Publication Data
A catalogue record for this book is available from the British Library

Library of Congress Cataloguing in Publication Data
Technologies of procreation: kinship in the age of assisted
    conception / Jeanette Edwards . . . [et al.]. – 2nd ed.
        p.   cm.
    Includes bibliographical references and index.
    1. Artificial insemination, Human–Social aspects. 2. Kinship.
3. Human reproduction–Social aspects. 4. Artificial insemination,
Human–Law and legislation–Great Britain. I. Edwards, Jeanette,
1954–   .
HQ761.T43 1999
304.6'32–dc21   98–35025
                                                                          CIP

    ISBN 0 415 17055 9 (hbk)
    ISBN 0 415 17056 7 (pbk)

Contents

Contributors

Jeanette Edwards is in the Department of Sociology and Anthropology at Keele University.

Sarah Franklin is in the Department of Sociology at Lancaster University.

Eric Hirsch is in the Department of Human Sciences at Brunel University.

Frances Price is in the Faculty of Social and Political Sciences at Cambridge University.

Marilyn Strathern is in the Department of Social Anthropology at Cambridge University.

Preface and acknowledgements

In 1989, while our group was preparing its research plans, Janet Finch published her appraisal of family obligations and social change in Britain. She asks about the kind of support that flows between family members, what kin relations are most crucial, and where feelings of obligation come from. Her answer to the last includes the way people appeal to 'blood ties' and the bond of 'flesh and blood' and thus to the facts of life. 'Biology seems to be the foundation of social obligation', and most obviously in the case of parents and children where offering support is regarded as 'just part of human nature' (Finch 1989: 36–7). As she observes, the idea that certain actions are determined or required by biology is important not because it is true but because of the meaning this gives kinship.

In the British context that Finch describes, kin relationships are being presented in terms of a special connection between social relations and natural relations. This is what gives them significance. The connection does not depend on the circumstances under which persons appeal to it or for that matter discount it. It exists as a mode of thinking about the foundation of relationships, and thus exists as a cultural reality. So the connection is there whether or not it is used to drive home an obligation and whether or not it is open to dispute. Indeed, part of the force of the biological idiom lies in its reference to an immutable condition of human life that has to be taken into account in people's social arrangements. With respect to those who appear in this book, it is taken into account in their ideas about the manner in which ties of flesh and blood, especially between parents and children, are formed through procreation. For many of them, procreation is not just about how human beings come into being – it is also about how relationships come into being, and relationships that have an influence not just on early life but throughout a lifetime. Inevitably, therefore, changes in procreative practice will have repercussions for thinking about the formation of such relationships.

Also in 1989, the British Parliament was debating the Human

Embryology and Fertilisation Bill. Legislation addressed one of the outcomes of recent developments in reproductive medicine: the need to regulate 'the use' of human embryos. The embryos that were the special focus of legislation were those that new procedures in the treatment of infertility had created outside the human body; the bill also dealt with donated gametes (ova and sperm). There was much talk, both within Parliament and outside, of what were colloquially called the 'new reproductive technologies' and what these new technologies meant for individual lives and for society at large. Debates turned on how far they were of self-evident benefit and what limits should be put on 'interfering' with 'nature'. Members of the scientific community expressed regret that the public often tended to run together all kinds of futuristic scenarios that impeded appreciation of both the extent and the limits of what scientific research could accomplish. It had been earlier feared, for instance, that such scenarios blocked the 'better understanding of infertility, contraception, birth defects and genetic disease' that support for embryo research would bring (*New Scientist* editorial, 8 December 1987). Concurrent with such concerns, the Economic and Social Research Council had had a research initiative on 'The Public Understanding of Science' under way since 1986.

Public depiction of the new reproductive technologies involved 'understanding' what exactly interventions in biological processes could or could not do; it also involved 'understanding' the kinds of connections to be drawn between natural and social relations. There were members of the social science community who regretted that more research had not been directed towards investigating the social implications of the new technologies. Sarah Franklin and Frances Price contributed to an early overview of social issues at the British Sociological Association annual conference in 1987 (McNeil *et al.* 1990), the year that Michelle Stanworth's (1987) edited collection also appeared. Margaret Stacey reiterated the regret at the British Association for the Advancement of Science meeting in 1990 (see Stacey 1992). In the United States the 'gap between cultural values and medical technology' in this area was first addressed at the American Anthropological Association meeting in 1985 (Whiteford and Poland 1989). While these are the beginnings of social science enquiry, and join a burgeoning literature on ethical, legal, feminist and other discussions, the history of research in this area is still brief.

When HMSO published the results of a national study of triplet and higher order births in 1990, this was the first population-based investigation of the problems faced by those responsible for the care of these children in Britain (Botting *et al.* 1990). Its co-authors included Frances Price, who had also been involved in the first phase of The Public Understanding of Science' initiative. The research had been instigated because an increase in multiple births evident in national statistics was believed to result from an increased use of fertility drug treatments and from procedures for assisting conception. The consequences for the parents of four or five babies born simultaneously are spelled out in terms of the practicalities of the parents' lives, and the report left no doubt about the palpable and long-lasting effects of certain fertility treatments. There was also the immediate impact that such treatment might have on intending parents, as Sarah Franklin was discovering in her investigations of the experiences of women who had sought or undergone in vitro fertilisation (IVF) (Franklin 1992). These people found their lives changed by the possibilities of fertility treatment in ways – both positive and negative – they had never imagined. In both cases, some of the implications for those directly involved with the new reproductive technologies were made evident.

Yet such persons (parents of triplets, say, or women undergoing IVF treatment) will always be in the minority in a population, and their circumstances seem very specific. Moreover, they come into contact with the services offered by reproductive medicine by seeking assistance to problems they already have. In what sense is 'society' at large affected? However concrete and palpable the effects on individual lives, what does it add to talk of 'social' implications? In order to consider this question, the authors of this book formulated the project on which it reports, and became for that purpose a research group based at Manchester University. They wished to ask what a social science enquiry might mean in this context, and in particular what social anthropology could contribute.

Social anthropology comes into the picture for one very good reason. The subject has always had a special place for kinship in its theoretical apparatus, and if procreative practice were about anything, it would seem to an anthropologist to be about relationships of kinship. Kinship offered a focus: one could consider social implications in terms of the implications for kin relationships.

If this seemed self-evident to Marilyn Strathern, it was because she was, in 1989, writing about current reconceptualisations of kin ties, both within anthropology and in terms of 'English' folk models (see Strathern 1992a). At the same time, she was aware how unready the anthropological community would be if it had to respond to specific questions about the social entailments of new reproductive possibilities. She had been put on the spot by one such enquiry concerning egg donation between relatives which came from the then Voluntary Licensing Authority in 1987. There were no anthropological investigations to which she could point – certainly nothing comparable to Robert Snowden's (see Snowden and Mitchell 1981; Snowden *et al.* 1983) long-term research with those involved with donor insemination or Alexina McWhinnie's (1967) earlier case studies showing the effect of adoption on perceptions of family life. There was Peter Rivière's (1985) commentary on the Warnock Report (followed by Cannell 1990; also Abrahams 1990), but even in terms of general anthropological interest in kinship there was little recent material. Jean La Fontaine's (1990) concern with child abuse provided one of the few anthropologically informed studies in Britain. From the double perspective of philosophy and anthropology, a synthesis of 'Kinship and Marriage in England' appeared in 1987 (Wolfram 1987), and particular aspects of kinship had certainly received detailed attention (e.g. Charsley 1991; Wallman 1984). However, nothing in recent years had displaced the comprehensive and first-hand work of Raymond Firth and his colleagues in London (1969).

If anthropologists were unready in one sense, they had acquired certain expertises in other aspects of British life. Jeanette Edwards, for example, was completing an ethnographic study of ideas of identity and relatedness in a north-western town (Edwards 1990). Here kinship was one among several contexts for the way people thought about themselves. And it had been in the context of ethnographic enquiry into other concerns that kinship most often appeared in anthropological analysis (e.g. Cohen 1987; Okely 1983). Thus the topic figured in accounts focused on ethnic communities (e.g. Ballard 1990; Bhachu 1985; Saifullah Khan 1977; Werbner 1990; also Benson 1981), and research on West Africans in Britain had included a pioneering investigation into fostering (Goody 1982). It was clear that a study that took kinship in Britain as its domain of enquiry would have to be exploratory.

The ESRC funded a project (1990–91) under the title 'The Representation of Kinship in the Context of the New Reproductive Technologies', and the research group came into existence for that year. It consisted of Edwards, Franklin, Hirsch, Price and Strathern, each of whom devoted from three to six months to their own part of the research. The time-scale necessarily imposed a methodological limit on our ambitions. Here Eric Hirsch's current investigations were suggestive. He was engaged in another ESRC study, part of the Programme on Information and Communication Technologies directed to the use of domestic technology among families in south-east England (Silverstone and Hirsch 1992). In listening to people contextualise their habituation to and deployment of such technologies, he was gaining information of a very specific kind: the cultural models through which views were explained. Cultural analysis affords one kind of purchase on the issue of social implications.

There were further reasons for thinking in terms of such an analysis. If what delimits kin relations and marks them out from all others are the connections people make between social and natural relations, these connections are of a cultural order. Attention to them might throw light on the very formulation of debate, as from different perspectives was also the hope of philosophers or thinkers concerned with technology policy, such as John Harris, David Lamb or Edward Yoxen.

The group undertook three exploratory studies, based on information provided by the parliamentary debates (Franklin), by ethnographic enquiry (Edwards) and by interview (Hirsch). Its own expertise was diverse. Franklin was an anthropologist through early training, but her study of women's experiences of IVF and their contextualisation by medical and media discourse was undertaken within the discipline of cultural studies; Edwards had carried out social anthropological fieldwork both in a north-western town, where she had resided for a year, and in a city-based voluntary housing agency; Hirsch, a social anthropologist whose first field was Papua New Guinea, had experience in development issues and had joined an inter-disciplinary research team in the domestic technologies study. Strathern was the only member of the group whose skills fell entirely within anthropology. She, like the others, depended much on the advice offered by Price, a medical sociologist, who acted both as consultant to the group and as contributor. Price's analysis from the point of view of clinical practice gives us our fourth study.

Several scholars have been individually named in this preface: they all provided help, encouragement and information in one form or another, some indirectly and others through direct conversation. Our appreciation is emphatic. In addition, the group benefited from a visit from Sheila Hillier and from the interest, each from their own perspectives, of Margot Brazier, Erica Haimes, Naomi Pfeffer and Gail Vines. Thanks are also due to those, drawn from a range of disciplinary backgrounds, who attended a one-day seminar held in Manchester in September 1991 and who responded so generously and with insight to the preliminary papers we presented there. We have drawn from their comments in this book, without separate acknowledgement but certainly to the book's enhancement.

M.S.
Manchester
June 1992

Note

The support of the Economic and Social Research Council is gratefully acknowledged. The work was funded by ESRC award number (R000 23 2537).

Introduction to the second edition

The authors

Kinship in the age of assisted conception has turned out to be a more thought-provoking subject than one could ever have imagined.

Why kinship? To a greater or lesser extent, part of everyone's identity as a person is derived from knowledge about their birth and about how they were brought up. It follows that such knowledge is also social knowledge, in that it presumes connection and relationship with others. Those others are persons with their own identities, so that kinship entails intimate participation in the way other people construe their identity too. Here, among different populations or at different times in history, birth, nurture, inheritance and diverse ways of maintaining relationships have all received different emphasis. The late twentieth-century development of the means to alter what many would have said were immutable processes of birth has created a new and complex vehicle for conceptualising connections.

The increasing visibility of outside assistance throws into relief the significance of birth over other ways of creating connections between kin. At the same time, that assistance changes the field within which such connections are mobilised and normalised. Those who in the past would have suffered infertility in silence, or turned to adoption, may feel they should be seeking out remedies for failure to bear children themselves. In so doing they act out new definitions of what it is to have one's 'own' child, and refigure the field of relatives. And the very procedures of assistance throw further into relief the significance of the means through which these ends can be achieved. For the people who are the subjects of this book, these means are both social – that is, comprising everything that goes into the practice or intention of bearing a child (what conceiving and giving birth 'means') – and also, importantly, technical. Seen as harnessing science, technical means frequently amount in people's eyes to a 'technology', and reproductive medicine is widely regarded as having become technology-enhanced. 'Assistance' of a technological nature which has the capacity to intervene in the lives of some has the potential of making everyone aware that procreation does not simply belong to the order of things. For those with access to the remedies which this enhanced reproductive medicine brings, and by access we include here having information about the possibilities it offers, the life-course may assume a new potential.

The result is twofold. First, in terms of those individual lives, choices exist that did not before: people make decisions about procreation in the context of an expanding range of possibilities. Second, the arenas of decision-making have proliferated: there are new domains and social actors involved, new alliances of medicine, ethics and law, not to speak of commerce, and thus new interests invested in the way people conceive of kinship. This book examines both dimensions. It offers insights into people's evaluations and judgements as part of the way in which they translate the possibilities of the 'new reproductive technologies' (NRT) into their own experiences. Yet 'people' never exist as generic entities: we are concerned with specific persons from specific locations. Within the compass of early 1990s England, these locations are deliberately diverse; they replicate a small part of the complexity of the field of identities, agencies, practices and interests which is redefining kinship.

I

Since 1993, the year in which *Technologies of Procreation* was first published, developments have proceeded apace. Reproductive and genetic technologies enlist not only human beings, but also other animals, as well as plants and micro-organisms.[1] They may even make explicit connections between reproductive futures across a range of life forms. In these intervening years, further possibilities for assisting human conception have in some cases proved too controversial to be taken up and in some too technically ambitious to put into practice (at least for the time being). Others have been heralded as welcome breakthroughs. All we would remark on here is the continuing accompaniment of anticipation and doubt. Public ambivalence has, so to speak, kept pace. Ambivalence was already evident in the early 1980s when the British Warnock Report (1984) was published, and was widely rehearsed again in 1989/90, a moment of unprecedented public attention in Britain stimulated by the parliamentary debates over the Human Fertilisation and Embryology Bill.

The anticipations and doubts of 1989/90 were then and have since been attributed to a conflict between 'traditional family values' and the advance of science. But to construe the whole issue as caught on the horns of that particular dilemma obscures numerous dimensions of social reality and ignores many of those who made their views evident. Ideas about tradition versus progress were certainly voiced but frequently only to air wider reflections, questionings and doubts; many found themselves in considerable difficulty in thinking through some of the social and ethical implications. The dilemma of tradition versus science/progress is a poor description of the level of public debate. This is what *Technologies of Procreation* begins to document. The fact that it is focused on kinship does not mean that it is focused on 'traditional family values'.[2]

On the contrary, it was clear to the authors at the time that if primacy were given to 'family values', traditional or not, it would obscure a whole matrix of intimate relationships of which the new reproductive technologies had become a part. The way we chose to address this set of affairs was to focus not on the institution of the family but on kinship. The concept of 'kinship' enabled us to address issues of relatedness without presuming particular institutional forms. This focus deliberately freed the study from the rhetoric of family values while still attending to the way in which people were making diverse arguments and counter-arguments relevant to themselves as parents and relatives – as persons who were involved, or could anticipate involvement, in one another's lives. That this involvement could be either positive or negative was as much acknowledged by clinicians and Members of Parliament as by anyone. If we neither demonise technological intervention nor romanticise kin relations, the same is true of most of our subjects. The book begins with problems voiced by a number of clinicians (who from the point of view of those seeking treatment, at least, are close to 'science'), and from there considers the manner in which a range of diverse others connected their hesitations to the realities of social relationships.

II

NRT shifts the study of kinship from the study of parents, children and other relatives into a wider domain, a complex field of human and technical relations brought about by another complex field, the mix of institutions, techniques, investments and markets, as well as occupational and professional alliances, which now defines reproductive medicine. But, then, social anthropologists never did imagine that kinship was only about kinsfolk – their studies elsewhere were always open to issues in political and economic life, religion and so forth.[3] Perhaps it is not surprising that it should be in social anthropology that kinship has made a recent and unexpected reappearance in academia, at least in Britain and the United States.

The term 'kinship' does double service. It is at once a field of study and the subject of study, both a way of organising knowledge and a set of human relationships. What has been happening in the academic field, and particularly in the discipline (social anthropology) which first developed the concept into a theoretical tool, turns an interesting mirror onto what has been happening to people's relationships with one another.

The last five years since 1993 has witnessed a burgeoning of academic interest in kinship studies. Whether this has been stimulated by the new legal negotiability of parent–child relations, by the publicity given to transactions in body parts or by popular accounts of the new genetics, the comparative study of kinship is firmly back on the anthropological agenda. Social anthropologists remember they have a long past in this area, in a manner reminiscent of the advent of feminist scholarship when anthropologists discovered they had always attended to the 'study of women'. Yet 'NRT' can no more be just added to older interests than gender relations could be added to topics entrenched in other paradigms. The argument of this book is that assisted conception is not simply another turn of a familiar wheel. That would overlook the very nature of the intervention which it brings into people's lives. The study of kinship through the lens of the kind of modifications prompted by reproductive technology will bring it into differently nuanced, differently defined, relations with other disciplines and interests.

In the words of Ladislav Holy:

> the new reproductive technologies and their discussion among spe-
> cialists and the general public have significant consequences for the
> anthropological study of kinship. The reason is that they bring clearly
> into relief the culturally specific Western assumptions about kinship
> which inform its conceptualisation and which have guided research
> into kinship from its very beginning.
>
> (1996: 25)

NRTs would certainly seem to have the potential to reconfigure the anthropology of kinship to the extent that its (anthropology's) paradigm was based on the formulation of kinship as the cultural construction of natural facts.[4] Yet their social power also exists on another scale altogether. It is simply not the case that present dilemmas produced by IVF and the like are 'a "problem" for the essentially "Western" (Euro-American) societies that have developed them rather than for other societies in the world' (Parkin 1997: 126). IVF, for example, is now widely deployed across the world. It has become in that sense a global phenomenon; whatever the original location and reasons for its development, diverse locations will find diverse reasons for its use. Reasons of the kind described in this book spring from certain Western preoccupations, some of which may be exported along with the technology. Other peoples, with other preoccupations, will find other reasons.

III

Between their several projects, the authors explicitly took on a dynamic of diversity. Somewhat after the event, George Marcus (1995) formalised the notion of multi-sited investigations. This has fuelled an agenda that is spreading rapidly through anthropology and cognate disciplines, gearing everyone up to do 'multi-sited ethnography'.

Diversity exists within, not just between, cultures. In Britain, Hirsch notes the 'circuit of culture' project which is producing a multi-volume set of books, each focused on a specific moment of an informational circuit. It is not trivial, even if it is commonplace, to say that kinship also occupies multiple positions in people's diverse universes. In retrospect we can see that the events of 1989/90 allowed us to capture aspects of English kinship thinking as they appeared – streaking comet-like – across several partially connected domains: households, the media, Parliament, clinics. We could not have carried out the study, in turn, if we had not been able to profit from the mixed benefit of social anthropological, sociological and cultural study perspectives. The project combined findings from different social quarters, then, and was to some extent 'cross-disciplinary' and 'multi-sited'. But it was also none of these things. There is a prevailing and reductive notion that multi-disciplinarity and multi-sitedness are somehow virtuous in themselves, by contrast with the project of the single ethnographer studying at a single site. Yet the accounts here are as much the result of lone ethnography as they are the products of a team of researchers whose ideas and enthusiasm influenced and inspired one another. They offer separate but interrelated perspectives which, together, point to the kind of cultural diversity, common concerns and complex internal layering to be found at any one site on which the reader chooses to dwell.

In 1993 *Technologies of Procreation* joined a small number of early anthropological analyses (British examples include Cannell 1990; Rivière 1985; Strathern 1992b) which perceived a connection between issues drawn from the field of reproductive technology and issues in the field of kinship. In this new edition, each of the authors has added an Afterword, but otherwise let their chapter stand as an indication of concerns at the time. As for these concerns, social scientists are interested in the nature of debate as well as with the topics under debate. And while a sympathetic reader commented that the book still felt remarkably fresh in its topic, through the Afterwords we have taken the opportunity to reflect on how some of the public arguments were, and how they are now, being conceptualised.

The original studies addressed the way in which ideas about kinship inform and influence understandings of NRT, and NRT informs and influences understandings of kinship. But there is more to the reach of these two areas than either of these particular connections. One can begin to demonstrate this by indicating where the studies have led each of the authors. Telling briefly of the authors' current research interests (and recent publications) will make explicit how these topics connect with other concerns.

Frances Price continues to be engaged by the concept of 'facilitation' in reproduction, particularly in collaborative ventures which involve transfers between persons, as in gamete donation. Price asks, what are the conditions under which people offer (or refuse) reproductive assistance? Furthermore, what are the conditions under which secrecy in such collaborative ventures is maintained or eschewed? *Sarah Franklin* has pursued the interface between NRTs and the history of kinship theory within anthropology. She has also turned her attention to changing definitions of life and death in work on frozen embryos and Dolly. *Marilyn Strathern* has developed her interest in the role of knowledge in Euro-American kinship thinking. This has taken her in two directions: the management of information (including 'kinship knowledge') under conditions of proliferation, and knowledge as a new subject for property (intellectual property rights) in the context of claims over persons. *Eric Hirsch* is drawing on comparisons between England and Papua New Guinea to think about the differing way in which things and persons are rendered into entities. He has become increasingly interested in what happens in Papua New Guinea when Western conceptions of resources, extraction and compensation contend with local concepts of land, person and transactions. *Jeanette Edwards* focuses on the way in which idioms of relatedness are mobilised in many spheres of British social life and not just that immediately recognisable as kinship. They are as apparent in the ways in which people formulate their views and feelings about places, pasts, communities, institutions and homes as they are in the ways in which they constitute families.

IV   SELECTED PUBLICATIONS SINCE 1993

Edwards, J. (1998) 'Donor insemination and 'public opinion': an anthropological perspective', in K. Daniels and E. Haimes (eds), *International Social Science Perspectives on Donor Insemination*, Cambridge: Cambridge University Press.

Edwards, J. (1995) 'Imperatives to reproduce: fertility in the light of infertility', in R. Dunbar (ed.), *Reproductive Decisions: Biological and Social Perspectives*, London: Macmillan.

—— (1998) 'The need for a "bit of history": place and past in English identity', in N. Lovell (ed.), *Locality and Belonging*, London: Routledge.

—— (in press) *Born and Bred: Kinship and New Reproductive Technologies in England*, Oxford: Oxford University Press.

Edwards, J. and Strathern, M. (forthcoming) 'Including our own', in J. Carsten (ed.), *Cultures of Relatedness*, Cambridge: Cambridge University Press.

Franklin, S. (1997) *Embodied Progress: A Cultural Account of Assisted Conception*, London: Routledge.

Franklin, S. and Ragoné, H. (eds) (1998) *Reproducing Reproduction: Kinship, Power and Technological Innovation*, Philadelphia, PA: University of Pennsylvania Press.

Hirsch, E. (1998) 'Bound and unbound entities: reflections on the ethnographic perspectives of anthropology vis-à-vis media and cultural studies', in F. Hughes-Freeland (ed.) *Ritual, Performance, Media*, London: Routledge.

—— (1998) 'New technologies and domestic consumption', in C. Geraghty and D. Lusted (eds) *The Television Studies Book*, London: Arnold.

—— (1998) 'Domestic appropriations: multiple contexts and relational limits in the home-making of Greater Londoners', in N. Rapport and A. Dawson (eds) *Migrants of Identity: Perceptions of Home in a World of Movement*, Oxford: Berg.

Price, F. (1994) 'Tailoring multiparity: the dilemmas surrounding death by selective reduction of pregnancy', in R. Lee and D. Morgan, *Death Rites: Law and Ethics at the End of Life*, London: Routledge.

—— (1995) 'Conceiving relations: egg and sperm donation in assisted procreation', in D. Pearl and R. Pickford (eds) *Frontiers of Family Law II*, London: John Wiley.

—— (1996) 'Now you see it, now you don't: mediating science and managing uncertainty in reproductive medicine', in A. Irwin and B. Wynne (eds) *Misunderstanding Science: Making Sense of Science and Technology within Everyday Life*, Cambridge: Cambridge University Press.

—— (1997) 'Match-making in the clinic: gamete donation and the management of difference', in A. Clarke and E. Parsons (eds) *Culture, Kinship and Genes*, London: Macmillan.

Strathern, M. (1994) 'Displacing knowledge: technology and its consequences for kinship', in I. Robinson (ed.) *Life and Death under High Technology Medicine*, [Fulbright Papers 15], Manchester: Manchester

University Press. [Abridged in F. Ginsburg and R. Rapp (eds), *Conceiving the New World Order: The Global Politics of Reproduction*, Berkeley and Los Angeles: California University Press, 1995.]

—— (1995) 'Disembodied choice', in L. Rosen (ed.) *Other Intentions: Cultural Contexts and the Attribution of Inner States*, Santa Fe, NM: School of American Research.

—— (1995) 'Nostalgia and the new genetics', in D. Battaglia (ed.) *Rhetorics of Self-making*, Berkeley and Los Angeles: California University Press.

—— (1995) 'New families for old?' in C. Ulanowski (ed.) *The Family in the Age of Biotechnology*, Aldershot: Avebury.

—— (1996) 'Enabling identity? Biology, choice and the new reproductive technologies', in S. Hall and P. du Gay (eds), *Questions of Cultural Identity*, London: Sage.

—— (1998) 'Surrogates and substitutes: new practices for old?' in J. M. M. Good and I. Velody (eds), *The Politics of Postmodernity*, Cambridge: Cambridge University Press.

NOTES

1 Through, for instance, genetic screening (Rapp 1987, 1995), the artificial life sciences (Helmreich), the human genome project (Hayden 1998) and cloning (Battaglia 1995; Stolcke 1998).

2 For example, according to Mulkay: 'The debate over embryo research in Britain involved a clash between two contrasting images of the future' (1997: 153) – scientists saw a future where childlessness would be alleviated and genetic disease controlled, while their opponents feared the undermining of 'traditional family values' and the damaging of 'existing social relationships'. In fact, Mulkay revealingly indicates that it was the scientific lobby which attributed to the traditionalists outmoded ('Frankenstein') views of the horrors of science. He implies that it was to the science lobby's advantage that so-called opponents did indeed occasionally deploy Frankenstein imagery.

3 In studies of Euro-American family life, such issues were either regarded as outside forces impinging on families or else were theorised in terms of patriarchy or intra-relational psycho-dynamics. (The household, on the other hand, has long been the focus of attention in terms of economic and political analysis.) Strathern (1992a) is an attempt within the confines of a cultural approach, to do for English kinship what anthropologists routinely do for kinship systems elsewhere in the world.

4 Reconfiguring is, of course, something that academic disciplines do all the time, and it would be possible to tackle the paradigm as a Euro-American model inappropriate for many societies in the world (as in the collection on *Cultures of Relatedness*, edited by Janet Carsten).

Introduction
A question of context

Marilyn Strathern

Reporting on a pregnancy announced on behalf of an Italian who will be 62 years old when she gives birth, the British newspaper *Today* (23 April 1992) drew on a new epithet for motherhood: 'Test Tube Mum'. Its tone was guarded. While the report included the courageous words of the woman who had been helped through eggs donated from a family friend and by the in vitro fertilisation of those eggs with her husband's sperm – 'We have wanted a child for almost forty years and never had one' – it headed the piece 'Fury as Doctors Breed "Orphans"'. The clinician who gave assistance is also reported as expressing doubts. A confident assertion that she was 'in good biological condition' is followed by his hesitation:

> At first I had no misgivings at all, but now I am beginning to have some doubts because of the relationship between the mother and child. She may be too old to take on the responsibilities of bringing up a child. When this woman is 75, the child will be 12 or 13.
>
> (*Today*, 23 April 1992)

A spokesman from a British IVF clinic bluntly voiced another concern: 'This is generation-hopping.' And: 'Because the technology existed, society needed to decide whether it should be used.'

Alongside innovations in reproductive medicine come innovations in the way people turn them to their own ends. In this instance, what is innovatory is not the desire (to have a child) nor its embodiment (the mother-to-be becomes pregnant with the assistance of procedures now well-established since the first 'test tube' birth of 1978). It is the stage in life at which this happens to her. The paper followed the story with a feature article the following day that reflected on how a 64-year-old might cope with a 2-year-old. The journalist (Gordon) put the issue into the homely context of what it was like to respond to the growing needs of a child over its childhood and teen years, opening with a personal comment on how she felt about being woken at 4.20 a.m. by the cries of her own baby.

And one wonders how many commentaries will open, as I have opened this book, with a provocative case history that simultaneously signals new ethical dilemmas and appeals to the human interest of experiences familiar, directly or indirectly, to everyone. One suspects there will be no shortage of good copy. Instant issues are created by putting one case into the context of others – as the *Today* commentary does with an allusion to a case also in the press at the time concerning the pregnancy by rape of a 14-year-old in Ireland and the ensuing debate over abortion. The year before, the national press had flared up over so-called 'virgin births' being asked of fertility clinics. That drama turned on women seeking artificial insemination in ways that made the question of their fertility beside the point: these were women who declared they had not had and did not wish for sexual relations.

The 'human interest' of such stories is one of the subjects of this book. But I use the journalistic phrase, with its slightly dismissive overtones, for a reason. The *representation* of that interest poses an interesting set of problems. There is general agreement that the new reproductive technology has implications, foreseen and unforeseen, for society. But how one demonstrates the significance of those implications is another matter.

PERSONAL OPINIONS AND PUBLIC OPINION

MacNamee, the clinic spokesman in the *Today* article, stated that 'society' must decide about the uses to which 'technology' could be put. In this formulation, the technology appears prior to whatever use society might wish to make of it. Technology and society are thus presented as two distinct domains: the formulation presumes an exclusive demarcation between those experts who develop and administer new medical techniques (the technology) on the one hand, and on the other the pool of people from which patients and clients come and the pool from which public opinion about the new techniques will also come (society). Yet to appeal to society is also to appeal to an entity that exists in the representation of a range of views and embraces multiple interests. From this perspective, it thus includes the opinions and interests of clinicians themselves. Quite aside from their expertise, clinicians, embryologists and other professionals involved in reproductive medicine have their own views about what they are doing. In any case, they may say that they are responding to public demand for certain services. They – and their technology – are in this sense very much part of society. That was one of the grounds of the 1990 legislation that sought to regulate research and clinical practice involving work with embryos and donated gametes. The development and deployment of new technology in reproductive medicine may be seen both as apart from the rest of society and as part of society as a whole.

This apparent paradox is a product of the way in which people represent issues of public interest, such as that raised by the 'test tube mum', with respect to the diversity of opinion they feel there must be. At the same time, to understand 'society' in terms of the diversity of concrete events or personal lives also seems to *reduce* its importance. The idea of society debating the ethics of parenthood (who, for example, shall decide suitability for treatment) has a scale to it that Gordon's account of being woken up in the small hours does not.

On such a scale, then, the concrete lives of individual persons seem a reduced order of phenomena. People appear preoccupied with the realities of their daily domestic and working relationships. Indeed, it is by virtue of such concreteness that such realities are regarded as specific to individual circumstances and views are taken as personal opinions. Society seems to encompass everyone, so that any one individual opinion always speaks for less than society as a whole. Yet the concrete particularity of people's differing circumstances can also appear as not encompassable at all, and the range of possible personal opinions outruns anything one might wish to gather together as public opinion.

The Warnock Report on Human Fertilisation and Embryology opens with a reference to 'our pluralistic society' and the observation that it could not 'be expected that any one set of principles [would be] accepted by everyone' (1985: 2). A pluralistic view of society as composed of a diversity of interests and personal experiences might suggest that social implications will be talked about in interest-based and experience-based terms. Thus the elderly mother-to-be is reported as speaking from her own point of view, and the clinical expert from another. If there seems a weight of expertise from the medical side, then the newspaper balances that the following day. The elderly mother's words are matched with those of a younger mother who starts by speaking to her readers on the basis of common family experiences. Human interest then becomes an angle on the story.

The particular genres into which reporting divides are illuminating in two respects. They involve a representation of the way individual views relate to what is thought of as society as a whole. They also remind us that we are dealing with formulations that belong to a specific culture. Ideas about plurality, diversity, the relationship between personal and public opinion, appeals to society in the abstract or to the effect of technology or to what is thought to have human interest: these are all forms of discourse that are culturally specific. Any serious accounting of the social implications of the new reproductive technologies would have to take this cultural dimension into account. There is more to what people say than the view they are expressing. But there is also more to a cultural view than the analysis of genres.

CULTURAL CONTEXTS

The newspaper *Today* published Gordon's article ('Can a 64-year-old mother cope with a two-year-old child?') under a photograph of an elderly woman and a little girl whom we are invited to see as grandmother and granddaughter. (Rather ominously they are blowing out candles on a birthday cake which from the number of candles must be an older person's, if not the grandmother's herself.) This was no doubt an allusion to MacNamee's observation about generation-hopping.

Like the image of coping with a 2-year-old (conventionally a tiresome age) full of energy (conventionally a view adults hold of children – given evidence to the contrary they are likely to goad children into activity), the question about generations belongs to a conventional set of ideas about relationships. The conventions in question belong to a particular cultural repertoire ('culture' for short). Let us designate this repertoire Euro-American; at its most extensive, it comprises the wider universe to which some of the British views already quoted belong. In this culture, generation is associated with age as part of a natural process. (Other cultures, where for instance polygynous family arrangements can mean that there is a great age span between siblings, may focus on generation as a matter of succession.) At the same time, more weight is often put on women than on men to manifest natural process. Gordon quotes the statements of a psychologist who observes that there is nothing untoward in men wanting children at 62, and adds: 'I see no reason why a woman shouldn't break through the biologic barrier and have a post-menstrual baby' (*Today*, 24 April 1992). To see biology as a barrier is a distinctive part of the Euro-American conventional repertoire. (Not all cultures present human enterprise working with and against nature in the way Euro-Americans do, or think of bodily process as belonging to a special domain as is imagined in the concept of biology.)

Yet the fact that people deploy idioms and summon images that belong to particular cultural repertoires is hardly cause for surprise. It is in the differences between (and thus the specificity of) idioms and images that an anthropologist would see the workings of cultural process in the first place. However, this book does not address cross-cultural comparison as it is ordinarily understood in anthropology. Its address is Euro-American. Between them, the chapters offer comparisons internal to this culture.

Comparative awareness is also cultural awareness. A comparative exercise throws into relief the kinds of connections that people make between different parts of their experiences. *How* those connections are constructed, the way facts and opinions are brought together, reveal possibilities and limits in forms of representation. They may also reveal ideas in context. Let me suggest what is 'cultural' in all this.

In following through the implications of being a 62-year-old mother, Gordon makes a connection with the kind of parenting that might be at stake – above all, running after a demanding child (the demanding child is a special representation of childhood). She thereby makes a connection, as the initial newspaper article itself did, with family relationships. She writes: 'Opponents of the latest test tube creation claim that it is unethical because Concetta and her husband might not live to see their child through to adulthood and that as such it is like "breeding orphans"' (24 April 1992). In making a connection between the woman's pregnancy and family life, she also evokes connections between people as persons in relationships. In short, she puts the new possibility of post-menopausal motherhood *into the context of kinship*.

Cultural convention shapes the making of such connections. In the way in which experts are drawn upon (the clinic spokesman, the psychologist), in conjunction with appeal to common experiences (being woken in the night), or between what is seen as a possibility (a post-menopausal baby) and what is seen as a barrier or limit (biology), ideas are being related to other ideas. When a whole set of issues are brought together, as various factors bearing on family relationships are being brought together here, then they create a discrete context. In turn contexts are made discrete by how they are demarcated and drawn upon. As a consequence, any one set of substantive issues may overlap with others, or nest within them, become encompassed by larger contexts or divide into smaller ones. And more than one context may be called into play, as when one becomes aware of shadow dialogues or sub-texts to what people are saying.

The way in which cultural contexts impinge on and derive from social contexts for decision-making, such as those described in Whiteford and Poland's book (1989), remains to be studied. Here we focus on the fact that a cultural context provides an inclusive framework within which multiple issues can be related to one another. What includes also excludes. Thus the important factor in the Italian clinician's mind was the medical fitness of the mother to bring the child to term; in Gordon's eyes, how one could embark on motherhood at such an advanced age knowing the demands that were ahead; and in the mind of MacNamee, the question of propriety in going beyond the natural limits of women's childbearing years. Each of them created a specific context for the issue in making certain connections and not others. Such creation has a communicative effect – makes sense to others, calls forth a response in listeners – because it also recreates sets of ideas that are already connected. Pre-existing connections offer possibilities for thinking about new ones.

Anthropologists are interested in the contexts that people create for themselves. They would say that culture lies in the manner in which connections are made, and thus in the range of contexts through which people collect their thoughts. Indeed, we could put it the other way round, and state that people cannot talk about their experiences or state their opinions without summoning some kind of context for their remarks. In doing so, they mobilise cultural forms, such as the genres of 'scientific fact' or 'personal experience', or the 'human interest' to which journalists feel they should draw attention. In so far as ideas are inevitably contextualised, that is, shaped through the forms in which they are expressed, all human activity has a generic cultural dimension. At the same time, cultural repertoires are differentiated from one another by the degree to which such forms appear distinctive; specific cultures afford people specific kinds of contexts.

Gordon and MacNamee both bring up kin relationships as a context for thinking through some of the implications of pregnancy in elderly women. 'Kinship' works as a cultural context of the generic kind in so far as it provides a framework. But then so would 'medical progress' or any one of a multitude of frameworks; the point is that there is always a framework. 'Kinship' works as a cultural context of the specific kind in so far as it mobilises a particular range of ideas about human affairs. Certain experiences are attributed to relationships enacted through family life, but while these may apply to many people in modern Britain, they would not apply everywhere. There is certainly a distinctiveness about the role that biology plays in these formulations.

Our studies suggest that, for the modern(ist) and Euro-American culture with which this book is concerned, kinship affords a context in which people readily conceptualise the *relational* dimension of their lives. It is, of course, by no means the only one, though it furnishes metaphors for others ('family', 'brotherhood' and so forth). But it carries special meaning within this culture in so far as such relations are thought to have their foundation and rationale in the very conditions of coming into being, the procreation and nurture of human beings, and thus in the facts of life. Moreover, 'kinship' evokes the relational rather than the institutional aspect of people's interactions as is contained in the concept of 'family'.

What is at issue is less the kind of unit that a family may form than the fact that kinship constitutes a matrix of relationships. So when they act as kinspersons, persons are acting with others in mind. One cannot be a mother unless there is also a child; one cannot be an aunt or uncle by oneself. Strictly speaking, this is a generic dimension of relationships rather than kinship as such (it would be true of any mutual relationship), but relations of kinship carry a specific and double resonance for Euro-Americans.

First, such relations are particular: each person has his or her own constellations of kin and, metaphors aside, these are not generalisable to other areas of social life. They thus appear as concrete, intimate and personal. In this sense, they may even be regarded as set apart ('private') from the rest of society. This separateness becomes manifest in an element to which I have already referred. Second, then, is the extent to which kin ties are thought to exemplify biological or natural necessity. Biology (or nature) appears as a domain of its own. To understand how 'kinship' could be thought of as somehow apart from the rest of society will require understanding the domaining effect of such further contextualisations. This is one of the tasks of the accounts that follow.

In the meanwhile, we take kinship itself as a context that works in this culture to signal an interpersonal element in people's dealings with one another. In so far as this relational awareness is in fact also a social awareness, it thus makes explicit one of the social dimensions of life. So when someone considers the new reproductive technologies in the context of kinship, we would argue that he or she is offering a comment on their social implications.

THE FOUR STUDIES

It is no surprise that anthropologists drawn from a Euro-American background should think that kinship might prove a profitable domain within which to explore some of the social implications of the innovations offered by reproductive medicine. This was the starting presumption of the studies that follow.

Exemplary versus representative status

'Euro-American' applies to a population that is both larger and smaller than that of the British Isles. Even if one might think of there being a British society, there is no single British culture. Britain's inhabitants may share much that is distinctive in their outlook on life with others in Europe or North America (the larger Euro-American universe), but they may by the same token share much with others in South Asia, the Caribbean, West Africa or wherever (not all Britons necessarily subscribe to a Euro-American outlook). Add to that class or regional differences on the one hand, and international cosmopolitanism or self-announced sub-cultures on the other, and identifying a common culture becomes absurd. But one does not need to do so in order to identify distinctive repertoires of idiom and genre and distinctive ways of making connections and creating contexts. (The degree to which kinship is regarded as set apart from the rest of society, for instance, may well be a non-continental version of Euro-Americanism.) The four studies that are the core of the chapters which follow present clear commonalities and differences in cultural form.

In each case people would for the most part be able to make assumptions about what is meant by kin or relatives without themselves having to take differences of ethnic or regional origin, say, into account. If they all met, we think they would understand one another. Their understanding would be based on certain fundamentals that they would take as the obvious and majority view of the world. However, they themselves would not necessarily recognise the name 'Euro-American'. We need some further cultural designation for the specific presumptions, sets of ideas and practices that belong to the kinship system discussed in these chapters. No adequate term exists. 'British' will not do, for, in addition to the qualifications already entered, it refers in the first place to a population (rather than a cultural repertoire) and its citizen status. 'English' on the other hand is parochial (what about Scottish and Welsh?), hegemonic (elides a common tongue with a presumption of common habits and customs) and less clear-cut than an ethnic or religious category (such as Chinese or Sikh). Parochial, hegemonic and ambiguously bounded: perhaps this is exactly the set of connotations that will remind us that we are dealing with cultural facts. In that case, whatever their backgrounds, and whatever else they speak, in matters to do with kinship the people in this book speak an 'English' version of Euro-American. In this they are party to what *they* probably take to be a majority view in Britain. Certainly they are likely to be responding to the kinds of representations of the world that dominate the media and shape public information on the new reproductive technologies. English Euro-American is, in any case, the universal language of the professions and of legislation in Britain.

The studies are drawn largely but not exclusively from white British society and across a class range of persons, from housing tenants to the House of Lords. But they speak for no social categories. The studies do not aim to be representative in class, regional or ethnic terms, nor in terms of family experience for that matter. They were set up to elicit diverse data: in this each has *exemplary* status. Each study affords a recognisable example of the kind of contexts in which (personal and public) opinion may be aired. Between them they demonstrate both the limits and the possibilities of kinship as a context for reflecting on the social implications of the new reproductive technologies.

By playing down the class affiliations of the people whose views we studied, and by ignoring ethnic diversity, among other things, we wished to focus on other reasons for the kinds of perspectives people have. We also wished to make a point about 'majority' culture. Culture is not something that belongs only to minorities. It is there in the way clinicians set about explaining their task to others, or parliamentarians debate the meaning of fertilisation, as it is there in the way family members think about what assisted conception means for relations between in-laws or individuals compare the advantage of fertility treatment to adoption. It belongs, in short, to their discourses. This is true whether these are discourses delivered by experts or the lay public. What emerged as a commonality across the instances we investigated were certain (commonsense) assumptions about the constitution of kin relations. These assumptions in turn comprise a majority view in so far as the view includes the way 'other cultures' ('minorities') might be measured by their divergence from it.

Internal diversity

The studies offer four diverse contexts in which the implications of reproductive innovation have been discussed. While we may consider the language of each an English exemplar of Euro-American, each is also bound by its own specific conventions, by what it is possible to say, by what are taken to be the critical points at issue.

Two of the contexts were ready-made; that is, they already existed as domains of discourse among professionals who have their own language for talking about their work (Chapters 1 and 4). Two were created by our study, which set up the framework for discussion and elicited responses within its terms. These addressed persons whose knowledge of reproductive technology was lay rather than professional: respondents were simply drawn from different geographical areas (Chapters 2 and 3). From one point of view, there was no demographic overlap. It was as unlikely for someone to be a professional in both fields as it was unlikely for someone to live in both of the areas. However, from another point of view, the criteria did not demarcate exclusive sets of persons. The difference between professional and lay is not a difference between populations but a matter of the contexts in which persons apply expertise. An individual who is a professional in one area of expertise is bound to be lay in relation to other matters. At the outset, the professionals in this study were taken to be those whose work brought them into contact with reproductive technology. As we shall see, knowledge about kinship is also expertise of a kind, though it was very variably drawn upon.

Members of the research group brought a modest diversity of disciplines and interests to the studies. Rather than submerge these, however, they made them explicit in discussion. One of their common tasks thus became how to connect their different perspectives and their differently assembled findings. In this, the method of study replicated a significant dimension of the field of study: 'internal' cultural diversity. In some respects their findings reinforced difference; in others revealed unexpected convergences.

In giving an overview of recent innovations in reproductive medicine, *Frances Price* comments on the perceived urgency with which clinicians find themselves coping not just with new techniques but with new expectations on the part of those who seek help (Chapter 1). The clinicians are professionals in the area of fertility treatment. They are concerned with the development of techniques in so far as these directly affect the services they can offer; they are also concerned with the needs of those who seek assistance. Price draws into view a range of observations that consultants and clinical practitioners make about their work in this second regard.

Over the course of visits to and interviews with those working in ten clinics offering assisted conception, and over the course of other conversations, Price was made aware of what could be called a kind of shadow dialogue. Beyond the medical opinions that consultants might have, or beyond the exercise of professional discretion in their treatment of specific cases, could be heard a running commentary on the difficult positions in which clinicians sometimes found themselves. Similar concerns can be found in the professional literature. In brief, clinicians were having to make decisions about issues that could not be reduced to medical or remedial matters. Some expressed a quizzical or even anxious concern about the judgements required of them – for what some found unproblematic others found very problematic indeed – particularly over people whose non-medical circumstances raised questions about their 'suitability' as parents. Age and post-menopausal pregnancy raised such questions. Sometimes these concerns were handled with the confidence of the expert. But at other times clinicians made it evident from their comments that they were going beyond their domain of expertise.

By itself, each comment on its own might seem no more than a personal opinion – like the misgivings that the Italian IVF clinician admitted, second thoughts on how he had acted in that specific case. But in bringing together those comments that raise queries about expertise, judgement and 'how far' such techniques should go, Price gives them an identity. She suggests that these constitute a body of concerns about limits.

The concerns have one general feature: at their heart is a question about the area that professional expertise covers. While some may see no problem in making judgements of all kinds, others express reservations. They regard themselves as venturing into social matters, or matters at least that, as MacNamee said, society should pronounce upon. Yet this area has no other name. I refer to these concerns as a shadow dialogue in order to point up the manner of their constitution. They exist as hesitations or qualifications, as second thoughts, as facts perceived to be on the margins of clinicians' competence. They do not emerge as a clearly demarcated domain.

Prompted to think about the new reproductive technologies in the context of kin relationships, the people interviewed by *Jeanette Edwards* (Chapter 2) had no problem about demarcating a domain of concerns. Indeed, whereas Edwards had initially assumed that she would have to raise these issues in an indirect way, she found herself being overtaken by the readiness with which many people were prepared to extrapolate. Hypothetical conjectures about gamete donation or surrogacy led into the consideration of practical problems and concrete situations. Issues were translated into their consequences for relationships of all kinds.

Edwards spoke with residents of a small town in the north-west of England ('Alltown'), and of diverse social backgrounds within the relatively narrow compass afforded by the town itself. None of them had had occasion to seek IVF or similar treatment. But Edwards argues that they are not representative of any particular 'type' of lay opinion; rather, they exemplify some of the responses people may make when kinship becomes a reference point. She goes further, and suggests that in effect kinship was serving as a source of expertise.

Alltown residents were very clear about the importance of making connections between different areas of their experiences. The relational view of human existence that they propounded in this context was not simply a reflex of Edwards' questioning: they enlarged and elaborated on her questions with vigour. There was nothing vague or diffuse in residents' acknowledgement of social consequences. People set abstract scenarios about reproduction into the context of concrete family relations, drawing parallels with familiar experiences such as adoption. Nor did they stop at visualising the immediate consequences for parenthood, as Gordon did in talking about her experiences of motherhood, but referred to a whole range of issues to do with the ramifications of kinship, between affines, across generations, and so on. In the course of doing so, Alltown residents enunciated certain explicit values, such as the importance of individual uniqueness, the significance of knowing one's links in order to be placed, and expressed doubts about the limits to which links could be stretched or displaced.

Interested in the way people contextualised their observations about innovations in reproductive medicine, Edwards limited her own questioning. After the initial introduction of certain topics, she hoped that the conversations with her would develop as colloquially as possible. Her acquaintances did, after all, come from people she already knew, a pool of some 30–40 persons with whom she was on fairly intimate terms; conversations took place in different environments (kitchens, pubs), alone or in groups. She thus felt she had latitude to act as a conversationalist herself, though never disguised the fact that she had a special interest in the questions and answers. She was not the only person with a special interest. One of their own sub-texts was the kind of place that Alltown was and what it meant to belong, for matters to do with kinship bore on how much people felt part of Alltown or not.

Eric Hirsch embarked on a rather different study of lay views (Chapter 3), with a small number of couples living both in and outside London whom he had interviewed extensively on previous occasions. He saw all of them in a similar environment (their homes) and number (always as a male/female couple). In terms of family set-up and parenting experiences, however, these couples were quite diverse.

Hirsch initially introduced questions in the way that Edwards had, but then followed a sequence of topics that was held constant for all the interviews. Whereas Alltown people were free to draw on whatever relationships came to mind, these couples were in the position of having to deal with their own relationship there and then. This did not necessarily mean that they spoke as a couple, nor that everything that either of them said was spoken in the voice of a partner. But Hirsch suggests that, whatever else was going in his dialogue with them, the fact of the relationship was a presence during the interview. It therefore had to be negotiated in some way or other. He suggests this conjugal sub-text put limits on the way topics were discussed.

Some couples felt free to extrapolate in general and abstract terms about the kind of society they thought the future would bring. Indeed, some spoke as though it were up to 'society' to set limits; certainly they thought that society would be affected, and it would show in the quality of individual life or the morality of consumer choice. By doing this, they were, Hirsch argues, putting the implications of technological innovation into a relational context that included the 'relationship' between individual and society. The future of that relationship concerned them. Such speculation about the future was largely unprompted; a spontaneous translation, one could say, from the concrete issues of conception and birth to abstract images of the kind of society that people's choices could create. The nature of this society would affect the nature of parenthood.

In being willing to speculate on the future, these people attached to future possibilities the same range of positive and negative feelings that they did to the possibilities of reproductive technology. If they were guarded, perhaps it was because in thinking about the changes ahead, and the kinds of limits on change that might be desirable, bringing in the possibility of society changing also brought with it the idea that limits themselves can change.

The future was specifically in mind in Parliament's passing of the Human Fertilisation and Embryology Act in 1990. In the debates that led to legislation, Members of Parliament were simultaneously a professional body with a job ahead of them (taking decisions that would determine future regulations) and lay persons (mediating between the scientific community and the public). Hence the largely agreed-upon facts produced by scientific investigations were set alongside the diverse opinions that were known to divide the public. Chapter 4 considers how the new reproductive technologies, as they bore on the matters that came under the Act, were accordingly contextualised by members of the House of Commons and House of Lords.

Although, as in the other studies, *Sarah Franklin* was interested in what people had to say, far from being in a situation of asking questions, she restricted her analysis to the questions that the parliamentarians asked of one another. The parliamentary debates are her text. We could say that the debates comprise a record of a discussion that is precisely about the social implications of innovations already under way in reproductive medicine. The stage was a public one, shaped by its own conventions, with Members of Parliament both constrained by the views they knew divided them and encouraged by the open vote to take a large view of their responsibilities. Many pointed to the fact that their decisions would affect the future, including the way in which future generations would be born. Scientific fact, personal experience and speculations about the future all entered their deliberations.

But whatever they might have done as individuals in other contexts, in this they barely brought in issues to do with kin relationships. There were allusions to parent–child relations, and members of the Lords were concerned with the genealogical record. But they did not spontaneously demarcate kinship as a specific domain. Franklin argues this was in part because of the primacy of place occupied by the figure of the embryo, and the extent to which it was treated as an individual entity. She then turns the argument around and suggests that one could see the embryo as a kinship entity in a new form. But if it were, it was not in the first instance represented relationally. The focus was on envisaging how new individuals might come into being, not on how new relationships might also be created.

Despite her best intentions to put the parliamentary debate into the context of kinship, then, Franklin found that she was having to adopt an unconventional view of what kinship might be. But the 'absence' of much overt reference to kinship raised a pertinent question about the very activity of contextualisation or domaining. People seize upon kinship issues much more readily in some contexts than in others. The question of where it is and where it is not important to discussion in this area is taken up in Chapter 5.

Between them, the four substantive chapters attempt to show how the cultural domain of kinship may or may not work as a context for the way in which people think about the social implications of new reproductive technology. They underline the fact that what is contextualised from one set of perspectives will in turn form a context from others. Kinship offers a context in which ideas about medical innovation can be collected. Yet as the last case indicates, not all discussions about the social implications provide a context for kinship. Suppose it were the new reproductive technologies themselves that were taken as our context? Chapter 5 reconsiders the evidence. It points to ways in which the new reproductive technologies do or do not draw people's attention to matters of kinship. The next section briefly sketches the cultural reasons for supposing there would be a connection at all.

PROCREATION

If, as a cultural domain, kinship furnishes a context in which English Euro-Americans think through some of the relational implications of their lives, it is not simply because kin relations provide a model for interpersonal relations. I return to the point that they do so because of a significant further element in the model. Kinship is a context in which Euro-Americans talk about relationships based on biology. Kin relations are regarded as created in the human necessity to procreate. And it is procreation that the new technologies assist.

The term 'procreation' implies the creation of offspring 'brought forth' from the body. Those whose views are presented in this book would probably take creation as encompassing the whole process from fertilisation to birth. A social event (involving a couple as sexual partners) is imagined as sparking off the biological development first of the embryo and then of the fetus. The creation of offspring is thus taken to be grounded in a composite of social and biological factors. But since the couple become parents only by virtue of the biological development taking place, the social recognition of their parenthood must follow the biological fact. This is a modern and twentieth-century view.

The priority that Euro-Americans, English or otherwise, put on the bodily process of procreation is rather special to them. Indeed, a point of debate in anthropology is that while everywhere social arrangements attend to the production and rearing of children, it is not the case that everywhere the facts of procreation are taken to be of prime significance. Where they are, then the circumstances of birth confer an identity on the child. Whether or not the relationships are consequently activated, for Euro-Americans there is no getting around the tie that exists with those persons whose genetic substances combined at the child's conception. This is taken as a fact of life.

Two consequences follow from this Euro-American premise. First, whatever relationships are involved in family life, the presumed fact of that tie of substance is there. Thus, in the late-twentieth-century colloquialisms with which we have become familiar, regardless of who the social parents are, it is axiomatic that everyone always has biological or genetic parents. Second, the facts of life provide a powerful rationale or foundation for the naturalness of family and kinship relations. Indeed, in so far as parents take on a social role as a consequence of the biological connection, there is a kind of layering to ideas here. Biological process as a set of grounding facts is not only regarded as prior to but as independent of such relations. Hence it is amenable to medical and other treatment on its own. In theory, the biological process of conception can thus be assisted without reference to the social identities of the parties involved, though in practice this may well turn out to be a contentious issue. Assistance thus makes visible the way two perspectives – biological and social – are connected to each other in relations of kinship. The point becomes doubly evident when new procedures introduce new procreative actors. Indeed, technology may create a separation between social and genetic parent that would not otherwise be tolerated.

Parenthood is, of course, realised in many ways, and we are used to adoption and other practices that specifically provide parenting in the absence of the biological tie. Other 'natural' aspects to family life also serve as foundational assumptions, such as the importance of the child's developmental needs. There is certainly more to bringing forth offspring than the accomplishment of conception and birth, as there is more to fetal development than genetics. The constitution of the social relations of kinship is, in any case, a field of its own. To take English kinship in its fullest 'social' sense one would have to consider relations built up through marriage, affinity and partnership, the conduct and quality of interactions, the interrelation of dependency and support, and the effect and obligations that acknowledgement of relatedness brings. From this view, one would be considering the many ways in which intimate ties are built up with reference to factors other than biological connection. Edwards' and Hirsch's acquaintances are fully aware of this dimension.

In the anthropological debate to which I have alluded, one long-standing contention concerns what it means even to demarcate a domain of relations as 'kinship'. Anthropologists generally divide into two camps. They agree about the variability of cultural representations but not about their manner of foundation. The first camp sees kinship as universally constituted in biology. The second uses the term for the reproduction of persons by persons as a social process. Thus the second camp finds interesting the stress some cultures put on nurture and feeding (rather than procreation) in creating substance, on the transactions that legitimate or confer reproductive identity (given by society rather than nature), even on death (rather than birth) as the final source of inter-generational definition. In this second view, such factors cannot simply be understood as arising from the way in which social relationships are variably built up out of and beyond invariant biological relations. However, the anthropological debate as such is constituted through the views of *both* these camps: the relationship between them, the relative weight of natural and social facts, plays out connections already evident in indigenous Euro-American kinship thinking.

The connections as Euro-Americans imagine them go two ways. On the one hand, kin relations are regarded as ultimately founded on procreation as a biological necessity. On the other hand, the social arrangements that provide the living, daily context for the procreation of children are given justification by reference to the natural facts. Their distinctive nature is represented in terms of universal and inevitable biological process. The biological facts of life thus serve to ground particular values associated with kinship.

This is very evident in the way English Euro-Americans appeal to 'blood ties' in justifying a sense of obligation they may feel to close relatives, or conversely discount the blood tie in cutting loose from the constraints of family life or in treating friends more closely than kin or in becoming a parent by other means. (The blood tie remains a grounding point even in being set aside.) Whether emphasised or ignored or bypassed, to think of kin as those people bound to one another through the necessities of procreation is to represent relatives in a specific way. From this perspective, everything that surrounds the act(s) of procreation bears on how people represent the meaning of being related to one another. Consequently, as far as the identity of the individual person is concerned, his or her biological origins remain a fact which never goes away. It is this set of cultural connections that shaped our enquiries.

As a consequence, the research group focused on the procreative dimension to kinship, and ignored a repertoire of anthropological materials on classificatory relations, social interaction, marriage and partnership, and the significance of nurture in the parent–child relationship. It would have been possible to draw on such issues in order to emphasise the 'social' character of kinship; in fact, we would argue, it is already there in ideas about procreation. So our focus is the emphasis Euro-Americans give to personal and kin identity via the facts of biology, and thus the cultural nexus between conception, sexual connection and individuality that is simultaneously reinforced and bypassed by the new reproductive technologies.

The NRT

In its largest sense, the new reproductive technologies could be taken to cover a whole apparatus of modern techniques, from contraception to changing medical practices surrounding birth. Those which we touch on here are all to do with one part of the procreative process – namely, conception. Technologies for assisting conception fall into a class of their own. Indeed, they offer an example of how cultural contexts are created: for such technologies include practices that themselves require no artificial intervention but have become recontextualised by the range of new possibilities. Clinicisation is also encouraged by new and realistic fears about the dangers of infection in the transmission of human tissue. We have followed the colloquial designation, the New Reproductive Technologies, in places underlined by the barbaric shorthand 'NRT'.

The principal possibility afforded by the NRT stems from the realisation that the fertility of intending parents can be bypassed by intervention in the process of fertilisation itself. Fertilisation outside the body (in vitro, in glass) has not only made it possible to monitor the process, it has encouraged the development of techniques for using donor egg or sperm without the complications of sexual intercourse with a third party. As Price describes, IVF thus stands (as a metonym) for all the possibilities that now exist for assisting conception. When people talk of the technologies in general, then, they usually mean fertilisation taking place outside the body (the 'test tube mother' is a reference to IVF), or to gametes (eggs and sperm) being donated by third parties or to women bringing to term children formed in part or whole from the genetic material of others. While many of these arrangements would not be possible without the development of collection and transfer techniques (IVF implies subsequent embryo transfer), it is the context of 'technology' that makes others thinkable as part of an overall package provided by modern medicine. But why 'new'?

What remains new about these procedures is not just the further development of means to improve the conditions under which conception may be assisted; they are still new, as Franklin makes clear, in their challenge to ways of thinking about procreation. Whatever other interventions confront family arrangements, interventions in the manner of conception put the facts of life into a new context. But the new context plays off old ones. It would be impossible to consider changes in procreative practice without considering the cultural fact that when Euro-Americans talk about procreation, they are also talking about one area of life (biological process) which provides the images and symbols, as well as in their view the substance, of another (social relations of kinship). In the 1989 Report on Reproductive Technologies to the European Commission, this is stated quite bluntly: 'We pick and choose among the biological criteria because we want to designate the couple who intend to bring up the child as the parents, rather than the donor or surrogate' (Glover 1989: 57).

So although the Italian in the *Today* story became pregnant through donor eggs and embryo transfer, and although her womb was made receptive through steroid drugs which (so the report went) manipulate the womb lining to make it think the ovaries are functioning, 'Now at last', she is quoted as saying, 'I can be a mother with my own child.' The significance she claims for that relationship is represented by her carrying a child to which she will give birth. For others, it might be represented by genetic continuity with the gametes, or for others again by the natural wish to have a child of one's body, a wish that is felt to be biologically driven even if it cannot be biologically realised.

A sub-text to what people say, then, is a connection that already exists, an 'old' context for bringing together different orders of fact, and one that turns on the status of biological process in the creation of kinship. This books explores that connection.

It is inevitable, therefore, that the book is also concerned with the process of representation itself. At the beginning, I suggested that the manner in which people put over many of their ideas created a problem in this regard. For when ideas are categorised as a matter of personal opinion, they seem to have no authority or interest beyond the perspective of the individual concerned. And in the area of reproductive technology, relational matters often appear expressed in personal terms. But if it is appreciated that 'personal opinion' is a cultural form of expression, with its own conventions, one can raise the question as to its categorisation with respect to other forms. As we shall see, such categorisations are crucial to the way certain issues get into or are excluded from debate. This in turn renders the process of representation crucial to understanding the place that such technology is seen to occupy in society.

In introducing this volume with a story culled from the popular press, I did not mean that press reporting should carry any special weight. It is an exemplar of a genre. The story and the article that followed were presented by the newspaper with all the conventions of serious journalism: the human interest to make a connection with the familiar, the dialogue created by asking for diverse points of view, the attempt both to evaluate and to balance opinion. Despite the extraordinary events, it becomes in that sense a very ordinary story. Indeed, any number of similar events could have illustrated the point. The point was to make explicit an ambiguity that runs through attempts to deal with the social implications of the new reproductive technologies. The NRT are held to affect people in very personal ways; they are equally held to have an effect on society at large. But these entail incommensurable orders of information.

The studies here are also exemplars: culled from different domains of social life, they collect together certain threads that run through reactions to technological innovation in this area. 'The people' who gave us our information do not fall into groups or categories – they and their views are diverse – and none of them represents 'the public'. As a consequence, their opinions are not to be explained by reference to some other (supra-) context, such as class or occupational background or childhood experiences, and the views expressed here have not been sampled to make them representative of such factors. This is true whether the people are clinicians or parliamentarians or residents of the north or south of England. Rather, the studies distinguish these people by the kind of context in which we elicited information from them. Specifying the different contexts in which our studies were carried out makes each study in turn intelligible as a body of information.

Kinship is a conceptual domain (a context) in which Euro-Americans make evident certain relational aspects to their lives, and specifically those relations constituted through procreation. That includes the way some relations are regarded as prior to others. In reflecting on the desirability of there being a limit to the number of babies born from a single sperm donor, the Sixth Report of the Interim Licensing Authority suggests that large clinics could go up to 20 'without increasing the chances of [sexual] relationships developing between people who are [already kin by being] genetically related' (1991: 51). Now there need be nothing mystifying in the concept of relationship. On the contrary, we find that what may well be mystified in public debate is the idea of 'the individual', whether the individual is presented as a client seeking fertility treatment or as the embryo that is created outside the body. In abstract terms, it seems possible to think of such entities as discrete beings. In terms of the concrete realities of living, however, individual persons only ever move in a matrix of relationships with other persons. Euro-Americans tell themselves that when they speak of parents giving birth to children; individual persons are born already related.

The people whose views are presented in the chapters that follow all touch on the facts of relatedness in one way or another. We have either deliberately elicited their responses with this cultural fact in mind, or else our account makes visible what otherwise exists in shadow form or is put to one side and screened off from other considerations. In representing some of the different ways in which concerns have been expressed, it has seemed important to preserve the sense of plurality against which they form their views.

1 Beyond expectation
Clinical practices and clinical concerns

Frances Price

Previously intractable causes of both female and male infertility can now be circumvented. The escalation of technologies to assist conception in the past decade has been accompanied by an expansion of what the Human Fertilisation and Embryology Act 1990 refers to as 'treatment services' to couples, very largely in the private sector of medicine. One commentator has portrayed the developments in this field of medicine as 'reproduction without sex but with the doctor' (Brody 1987). Another cautioned, 'The issues are so new that there isn't an agreed ethical tradition and so there's a danger that whatever practices doctors drift into become the norm.'[1] But the doctor who practises in this area of medicine is not the doctor of old.

Infertility clinics offering assisted conception hold out the prospect of a solution for problems which people are willing to pay considerable sums of money to address. Those women and men who seek such 'treatment services' by and large become consumers in a competitive market in which a 'good enough' pregnancy rate looms large. But there are crucial differences in the mode of delivery of these services, compared to that in other medical specialties. In ways which have yet to be explored systematically, doctor–patient relationships have been transformed: the classic (textbook) doctor–patient format is compromised. Not only does the focus on 'the couple' fundamentally change the one-to-one relationship presumed between doctor and patient, but 'the doctor' is 'partnered' also. Typically, the clinician (as the medical practitioners specialising in the technique of in vitro fertilisation and embryo transfer [IVF] and its analogues will be called in this chapter) is paired with a scientist (an embryologist). And there is a division of labour between them. The clinician who pioneered IVF, Patrick Steptoe, and the scientist Robert Edwards, published their account of their collaboration in *A Matter of Life: The Story of a Medical Breakthrough* in 1980 (Edwards and Steptoe 1980).

Working together in teams, then, clinicians and embryologists have developed techniques such as IVF, and analogues such as gamete intrafallopian transfer (GIFT), to provide new clinical services. An array of further options includes the micro-manipulation of gametes and embryos, the use of donor gametes, and the search for 'host-mother' or IVF surrogates. This chapter charts some of the expressed concerns of those who are developing and providing treatment services. The context of such developments is briefly outlined.

The politicians and policy-makers who were involved in drafting the legislation which culminated in the Human Fertilisation and Embryology Act 1990 sought scientific legitimacy for their decisions. This thrust the medical and scientific communities working in this field into a new, high-profile and political role. It was expected that they would provide a firm and authoritative input, the expert evidence. Yet the crafting of policy has been and remains a more elusive process than this implies. It turns not only on who is expected to make the decisions but also on what is to count as evidence when decisions are being made. There is social limitation on room for debate. As one sociologist of science has pointed out, the very development and not just the application of scientific knowledge is increasingly tied to policy situations in which incomplete knowledge is pressed into policy use (Wynne 1991).

Despite the passage of the Act, however, recent developments in the field of assisted conception have reaffirmed the crucial role of the clinician in both decision-making and as gatekeeper to the delivery of services. Their decisions gain authority emanating from a medical setting and may prove difficult to challenge (Price 1992). As they seek medical assistance and 'treatment services', couples can generally expect that their plans for pregnancy will be greeted as proper and respectable. Nevertheless, such plans may become transformed, and have unforeseen consequences, in a context in which clinicians are encouraged to provide whatever services are deemed to be within the ambit of medical competence. In some licensed centres, egg or embryo donation prior to IVF can now be offered as such a service.

Far more than the facilitation of pregnancy is at issue. The significance of assisted conception extends beyond the prospect of pregnancy, birth and associated clinical risks and uncertainties. Women and men shoulder new kinds of risk and uncertainty concerning their future relationships, particularly if there has been a donation or a multiple pregnancy. I focus on two areas of decision-making: the first is that of multiple embryo/egg transfer in IVF and GIFT procedures; the second is that of egg donation. The chapter draws from interviews with clinicians and embryologists working in the field of IVF undertaken between 1990 and 1991 in the course of a research project which focused on women and men attending infertility clinics (Price 1991).

THE CONTEXT: TIME PASSING, TIMES PAST

Most women who attempt to do so conceive within one year. However, increasing numbers of women are delaying attempts to become pregnant until their thirties. Their chances by then are demonstrably less favourable, as fertility in women is generally acknowledged to decrease with increasing age.[2] Older women may experience great distress when they confront difficulties with conception:

> You realise you're in your mid-thirties and all these books are around you telling you that your chances of pregnancy are diminished as each year goes by. I hated birthdays. I loathed birthdays. I was coming up to my 39th birthday. Each time you have a birthday, time is churning on. And there is nothing you can do. You just grasp all the time at straws and they just give way.[3]

Clinicians are well aware of the pressure of time passing on their patients and perceive urgency in the expression of their desire to remedy their situation. One IVF clinician remarked to me[4] that in his experience infertile women were 'some of the most impatient patients in the world'. He added that he found his infertility clinic 'much more stressful' than his general gynaecological clinic. He elaborated further:

> The infertility patient puts you under a lot of pressure. Their attitude – I mean I'll give you an example. There is one question you ask of all women first, or one of the early questions you ask of her. How old are you? And the woman will look at you and she'll give you an age. And you write down her date of birth and then you look at it. Before you finish she says, 'Well I'm 34 on my next birthday.' Now that is against women's basic make-up. What do they do? They try to keep their age down. The truthful answer to the question is 'I'm 33.' But they *always* say – they will always add a year on . . . Now that is an interesting point. And it starts, it is the tone of the whole interview. The tone of the interview being the fact that they are really saying to you, look, you know, I'm losing an egg every month, you know. I'm going to stop one of these days. For goodness sake get on and do something about it.

Between one in seven and one in ten couples in the reproductive population seek help in their efforts to conceive (Hull *et al.* 1985; Mathieson 1986). Among these couples are those whose inability to conceive remains unexplained after all the standard diagnostic tests. The incidence of such 'unexplained' infertility is unknown. No physiological or pathological cause can be found for their childlessness: it is a symptom, not a diagnosis. Moreover, there is some support for the idea that psychological stress factors introduce or exacerbate difficulties with conception (Edelmann and Golombok 1989). Systematic research into the psychosocial aspects of failure to conceive is comparatively recent (Morse and Van Hall. 1987).

Historically, both the investigation and management of infertility have been accorded a low status in medicine (Pfeffer 1992). In the United Kingdom, criticism of the poor provision and coordination of services is coupled with evidence of inadequate financial planning by health managers. Where services are provided, they have been reported to be of limited effectiveness (Mathieson 1986; Pfeffer 1987; Lilford and Dalton 1987; Winston 1991). However, public *expectations* and professional *perceptions* concerning the management of infertility have been transformed since the introduction of IVF and the proliferation of clinical services.

The pressure on IVF clinicians arises not only from the demand for the new array of services arising from technological developments in the field but also from an attenuated time frame for decision-making. One clinician explained:

> You see, in the old days, it [time] didn't really matter. Because you sat back and the attitude was, well, if you give nothing to the patient they'll probably get pregnant anyway . . . But now that you've got all this advanced technology, you're under pressure to get it under investigation fairly rapidly, come up with answers and tell the patient the answers, discuss what they mean, and take serious decisions about what you're going to do.

Decision-making, he said, used to take 'as long as a year, from question to answer'. Now 'it's all go up front'. He added:

> [P]atients who attend the infertility clinics generally are much better informed, very much better informed. They're sharper . . . so that's the pressure that is on.

The history of the science of this field indicates the extent to which the early pioneers of IVF foresaw what a demand there would be if their researches into the fertilisation of human eggs bore fruit. But many years of intermittently controversial animal research by a handful of pioneers preceded work on human IVF (Rock and Menkin 1944; Edwards 1985). The idea of assisting fertilisation by extracting and fertilising a woman's egg with sperm and then transferring it to her uterus was the subject of animated discussion following publication in the 1930s of work on the fertilisation of rabbit eggs in the laboratory (Westmore 1984). In 1937, an anonymous editorial in the *New England Journal of Medicine* entitled 'Conception in a Watchglass' speculated that the profession would be 'going places' were such to be achieved in a woman. The editorial concluded, 'What a boon for the barren woman with closed tubes!' Nor were the early pioneers of human IVF hesitant to promote conceptions of need.

Yet these pioneers, including Robert Edwards and Patrick Steptoe, were working in relative isolation. Yoxen surmises that they were taking a professional risk with their work:

> [T]heir experiments were not thought to be in the mainstream of clinical or biological research and periodically they faced considerable public or professional hostility. . . . By the mid-1970s the practical goal of transferring a fertilised human embryo back to the uterus . . . was being attempted by several research groups around the world. Whether and in what terms these experiments had been discussed with local ethics committees, or with comparable national organisations, is unclear. But it is striking that when in 1978 the first child was born after in vitro fertilisation, the Medical Research Council in the UK let its scepticism about the value and safety of this procedure be known publicly and declined to provide any research funds. As one might expect Robert Edwards still talks about this with thinly veiled rancour. In the US a major ethical review of the field was commissioned by the Department of Health, Education and Welfare. In the event no public funds became available for this field in the US.
>
> (Yoxen 1988: 29)

Lesley Brown gave birth in 1978 to her daughter Louise, the world's first IVF baby, after a single fertilised egg had been transferred to her uterus during a spontaneous menstrual cycle (Edwards and Steptoe 1980). The full range of instances when IVF would be proffered, and the changes in the procedure itself which were to follow, were not at that time envisaged. Robert Edwards, writing in 1980, remarked:

> Patrick [Steptoe] naturally finds it painful to have to disillusion patients who have not fully understood the implications of our work. It was embarrassing, for instance, for him to have to disillusion the occasional lady several years past her menopause that there was no chance of her becoming pregnant.
>
> (Edwards and Steptoe 1980: 212)

Only a few additional IVF conceptions occurred during the next several years. A procedure which seemed to have a pregnancy rate of less than 5 per cent did not encourage potential practitioners.

It was not long before this picture changed radically. The introduction of ovulation induction to enable multiple egg recovery and multiple embryo transfer was a particularly important development and was associated with a higher chance of pregnancy (Trounson and Wood 1984). The reported pregnancy rate rose, and IVF became more desirable as an innovatory clinical service. Yoxen conveys the changed climate:

> By the early 1980s it seems clear that professional attitudes were changing, and that obstetricians in many countries began to consider developing or buying in expertise in this area, in order to extend their technical repertoire. The existence of a few specialist clinics indicated a very considerable worldwide market for this service. As the success rate rose slightly, although they remain at around 10 per cent overall, so did the number of scientific publications. Furthermore in the UK several evaluations of moral issues raised by in vitro fertilisation were begun by professional bodies. All of these eventually endorsed in vitro fertilisation, including that from the Medical Research Council.
>
> (Yoxen 1988: 29)

GUIDELINES AND STANDARDS OF PRACTICE

In the absence of data from other sources about what can be realistically expected, members of the medical profession who have pioneered an innovative technology are encouraged to be at the forefront of decisions not only concerned with what constitutes 'adequate knowledge' about its benefits, but also with what should be promoted as good practice for its use. It is no surprise therefore that, in Britain, standards of practice that had been followed by the small handful of pioneers were taken up and became the basis of guidelines devised by the Voluntary (and then Interim) Licensing Authority (VLA; ILA). Charged with the responsibility of licensing, of constructing interim guidelines and of monitoring centres undertaking IVF, this review body was set up jointly by the Royal College of Obstetricians and Gynaecologists and the Medical Research Council in 1985. It was formed in the wake of the findings of the Warnock Committee (published in 1984) to fill a now perceived vacuum while legislation was awaited.

However, particularly after the VLA's decision to encompass the issues of both research and clinical practice, their guidelines met with opposition:

views about good practice differed. Before long there were on the one hand clinicians who complained that the guidelines compromised their clinical judgement and, on the other, heated criticism of colleagues' practices. By the late 1980s, differences of opinion among clinicians and between clinicians and the VLA about what was ethically acceptable and about what should be left to 'reasonable clinical judgement' had surfaced in public. How was 'success' in an IVF unit to be defined? How many eggs and embryos should be transferred in any one cycle? What incidence of multiple pregnancy was acceptable? Was it appropriate to sacrifice one or more fetuses in a multi-fetal pregnancy? Should egg donors be anonymous? (Price 1988). Monitoring of practice and its effectiveness remains a delicate issue. Members of one IVF team wrote a letter to the *Lancet* stating their belief that 'unless there are statutory powers, it is unlikely that clinics will be honest about their successes. Until this is achieved, a standard and efficient level of practice will not be widely available' (Fisher and Webster 1987: 273).

These public disputes provide striking examples not only of the problems of self-regulation but also of the limits of expertise in this field. The VLA felt obliged to revise and extend its original guidelines to censure certain clinical practices as a matter of public policy, and temporarily to withdraw the licence of one centre that persistently ignored its advice.[5]

The subsequent passage of the Human Fertilisation and Embryology Act in November 1990 marked the end of a regulatory hiatus since the publication of the Warnock Report had put infertility services firmly on the public policy agenda. The Act provides for the establishment of a statutory review body, the Human Fertilisation and Embryology Authority (HFEA), which is required by law to maintain a code of practice that will apply to all infertility clinics undertaking activities licensed under the Act. These activities include infertility treatments involving the use of donated gametes or the creation of human embryos outside the body, research on embryos, and storage of gametes and embryos (Morgan and Lee 1991). Even in its limited scope, it is regarded by some clinicians as an incursion into clinical freedom. Yet there has been disquiet that the assisted fertilisation technique GIFT – in which eggs and sperm are placed in close proximity to each other in a woman's fallopian tube – is not regulated by the statutory licensing authority (unless donated gametes are involved), because it does not involve the creation of an embryo outside the body. Clinicians, as well as members of the former ILA, have voiced concern about this decision (e.g. ILA 1991; Winston 1991). The responses from the Department of Health have all been to the effect that the legislation was explicitly directed towards regulating work with (and storage of) embryos and donated gametes. The HFEA is, above all else, a licensing body. It has to operate within the terms of the 1990 Act.

The issue of 'patient selection'

The question of which people should have access to 'treatment services' is a source of controversy. In Britain, all three publicly funded NHS units restrict treatment according to age; usually any woman over 38 will be refused treatment. One clinic refuses to accept women over 36 on to their waiting list. Clinicians justify the age policy by claiming that it is a fair criterion to use when distributing scarce resources simply because older women are less likely to become pregnant after IVF. They may cite the fact that pregnancy rates have been reported to decline sharply after the woman reaches 40 (Piette *et al.* 1990). Yet in the clinics in the private sector, where patients have to pay for their treatment, a different age criterion may prevail. Women in their forties (even those approaching 50) may be accepted on to the IVF or GIFT programmes.

In both the public and private sectors, however, the 'selection of patients' may also be linked to clinicians' judgements about who is 'suitable' for parenthood by virtue of their relationships. A late amendment to the 1990 Act, Section 13(5), states that:

> A woman shall not be provided with treatment services unless account has been taken of the welfare of any child who may be born as a result of that treatment (including the need of that child for a father), and of any other child who may be affected by the birth.

Neither the Act nor the HFEA gives guidance as to how this ruling should be interpreted. It becomes, in effect, left to the clinicians' judgement.

At the point of acceptance for treatment, both past and present relationships may be considered. Most assisted conception clinics restrict treatment to heterosexual couples who are either married or have been living together for a number of years. Few clinicians, it seems, are prepared to offer IVF to those with 'inappropriate' or absent relationships: in effect this means that treatment services are denied to single women or to lesbian couples. The IVF practitioner Winston (1991: 558) observed:

> Most medical practitioners are very reluctant to offer such women treatment, though they find it difficult to provide a rational reason for refusing. Anecdotal evidence is occasionally produced by physicians, suggesting that babies born to lesbian mothers may in some way be

disadvantaged and may suffer from the lack of a father figure as a 'role model'.

Winston believes that it is reasonable to get evidence of the 'safety' of such children first. He reflects:

> I, personally, am somewhat worried about offering IVF to single women, or those in lesbian relationships. Perhaps as long as such a small proportion of patients have access to what is a 'scarce' treatment, and when there are considerable waiting lists, we are justified in limiting these free treatments to couples in established 'family' relationships. And if we are not prepared to offer free treatments to such women, then we should, it seems to me, apply the same restriction in the private sector.
>
> (1991: 558)

He does not, however, hold that these restrictions should apply to all procedures intended to alleviate infertility:

> A lesbian or single woman with blocked Fallopian tubes must surely have the same right of access to tubal microsurgery as a married woman. Here treatment is designed to correct a disease process or change existing pathology. In a curious way, in vitro fertilisation is quite different, as it is not a treatment for the cause of infertility or the underlying condition, but a way of getting a person pregnant.
>
> (1991: 558)

There is a remarkable switch in perspective here.

By contrast, another IVF clinician, whom I interviewed in 1991, reflected a different view:

> There are so many people who bring up their children in a single-parent sort of situation. I feel very loath to apply rules to the infertile when the fertile don't have these rules applied to them.

He was reluctant to make judgements about 'suitability' for treatment:

> I mean who's going to, who *should* stand up and judge these people, you know? It seems a very hard thing to me, I'm afraid. I feel disinclined to be the person who does this.

He arranged for those women who told him that they wanted donor sperm because they had no partner to talk to the infertility counsellor. He was prepared to go ahead 'if we've got stable, sensible women'. He added, 'We've done it, you know, for years.' However, he told me of a recent request from a single woman that was still under consideration:

> This woman declared that she had got relationships but they were all rather unstable, and that she wanted a child for herself because she was frightened of being lonely in her old age. So she clearly wanted this child for reasons which were very intensely self-centred, and our counsellor was very anxious that the woman really wasn't mature enough to give this child a satisfactory parenting. And she [the counsellor] produced a whole list of risk factors which will give you disturbed children, basically, and she felt this woman would bring a child up in a very high-risk environment. We [the IVF team] are thinking seriously about whether we should be applying these sort of criteria to exclude people who have been particularly worrying.

At the moment there were no criteria used in his clinic to exclude women. 'I don't think we've ever excluded anybody actually,' he said. But added:

> We've had some, we've had one or two people who we've been in very grave doubts about. I will say that what usually happens to those people is that they don't usually stand the – it's quite gruelling IVF – and these sort of people with chaotic lives can't cope with the system and they fall out.

Rather than being selected by others as suitable for treatment, some people begin an IVF programme and then find themselves unable to comply: in effect, they screen themselves out. And sometimes this is because their relationships hinder their participation.

MULTIPLE EGG AND EMBRYO TRANSFER AND THE RISK OF MULTIPLE PREGNANCY

A crucial issue is the number of eggs or embryos to be transferred. When three or more eggs or embryos are available, three are generally transferred. This has come to be regarded as the norm, since most clinicians believe that this practice is likely to achieve a more favourable pregnancy rate than transferring a smaller number. Yet it is controversial because of the risks of a multiple pregnancy to both the pregnant woman and her developing fetuses.

In the early 1980s, Biggers (1981) encouraged the transfer of more than one embryo by suggesting that the IVF pregnancy rate would increase with the number of embryos transferred in each treatment cycle. Edwards (1985) later argued that an embryo capable of implantation somehow helps other transferred embryos to implant. He subsequently retracted this suggestion, but by the mid-1980s pooled counts from IVF centres around the world seemed to confirm such predictions and encouraged the transfer of between three and six embryos (Seppala 1985). Concern about the marked increase in multiple pregnancies came later, principally from another branch of medicine, paediatrics.

Annual statistics produced in the United Kingdom by the Voluntary and then Interim Licensing Authority for Human In Vitro Fertilisation and Embryology show a clear association between the rise of multiple births from 1985 onwards and the increased use of IVF, GIFT and associated procedures (ILA 1991).[6] Better access to ovarian follicles with ultrasound-guided retrieval, along with new combinations of ovulatory drugs, have enabled larger numbers of eggs to be collected. From 1986 onwards, neo-natal paediatricians voiced concern about the incidence, risks and consequences of multiple births, their effects on neonatal services and the cost implications for the NHS (Levene 1986; Anderson 1987; Levene 1991; Peters *et al.* 1991; Scott-Jupp *et al.* 1991). Most women undergoing assisted conception in the private sector transfer to NHS care once they are pregnant. Private clinicians thereby relinquish responsibility for these pregnancies to the public sector.

Since 1987, the Authority's guidelines have stated that no more than three eggs or embryos should be transferred in any one cycle unless there are exceptional clinical reasons, when up to four eggs or embryos may be transferred in any one cycle (VIA 1987; ILA 1991). Yet clinical practice varies widely. The ILA's Sixth Report states that 9.9 per cent of all IVF transfers in 1989 were of four or more embryos, despite the Authority's guideline that the limit of four embryos should be transferred in exceptional clinical circumstance only (ILA 1991). In the case of GIFT, the ILA Report (1991:18) informs:

> 59 per cent of all cases had four or more eggs transferred. This is of particular concern in that the transfer of five or more eggs resulted in a multiple pregnancy rate of 41.7 per cent without a significant increase in the pregnancy rate.

In March 1991, the shadow Human Fertilisation and Embryology

Authority (which formally had no legislative authority until August 1991) issued a document explaining the reasons and assumptions behind some of the provision in the HFEA's consultation document on the Code of Practice. The Authority canvassed views:

> Some people believe that there is no longer any justification for replacing even three eggs or embryos, and that the upper limit should now be set at two. We would be interested to hear views.
>
> (HFEA 1991: 20)

At least two licensed IVF centres in the UK are routinely transferring no more than two embryos per treatment cycle even when more than two embryos are available (Dawson *et al.* 1991; Waterstone *et al.* 1991). Another licensed centre utilises the woman's natural cycle with the intention of retrieving a single mature egg and subsequently transferring a single embryo without the use of ovulatory drugs. But in the Code of Practice published in August 1991, three embryos were stated as the maximum to be transferred in licensed centres. The Authority gave no public justification for its decision.

For most people, the prospect of triplets or more is too remote to be imaginable. Even with the rapid rise in the number of births of these children in England and Wales, only 28.6 sets were born per 100,000 deliveries in 1989 (compared with 12.2 per 100,000 in 1982). Ignorance therefore seems understandable: few know of the problems faced by those responsible for their delivery, care and welfare. Yet in the context of consent being given to procedures that increase the risk of plural births, lack of information becomes an issue.

In 1986, as the rise in the numbers of plural births became apparent in national registration data, and as paediatricians increasingly gave voice to their anxieties about the neonatal consequences, the Department of Health agreed to support a national study: the United Kingdom Study of Triplets and Higher Order Births (the National Study). It consisted of surveys of obstetricians, general practitioners, paediatricians and parents (Price 1989; Botting *et al.* 1990). A proportion of the parents were also interviewed.

The National Study showed that such children are, in all senses, high cost (Mugford 1990). Triplets and quadruplets are more likely than single babies to be of low birth weight and to be born prematurely, with all the associated neonatal difficulties and risk of disability and continuing developmental problems. Over half the quadruplets and just over a quarter of the triplets weighed less than 1,500 grams at birth. Births occurred before 32 weeks' gestation in about half the quadruplet or higher-order births and a quarter of the triplets. By contrast, information from the British Maternity Hospital In-Patient Enquiry indicates that only 1 per cent of singletons and fewer than 10 per cent of twins were born before 32 weeks. Furthermore, the National Study showed that 28 per cent of the triplets and 62 per cent of the quadruplets spent a month or more in neonatal intensive care. Mugford (1990) calculated that the average National Health Service cost of hospital care was about £12,000 for triplets and more than £25,000 for a set of quadruplets or more. Neonatal care accounted for more than 60 per cent of the total cost. And very few parents in the UK seek to pay for neonatal care in the private sector of medicine.

When the children come home from hospital, their caretakers face a further and very demanding situation. It is not possible for one person to cope alone for any length of time (Price 1990b), and where space is confined, it is likely to become an issue of great consequence (Price 1990c). Reported difficulties were emotional as well as practical. Familiar time-tables, as well as relationships, were disrupted. Seldom were these consequences anticipated. The situation described by parents was far from normal. Indeed, attempts to behave 'as normal' usually had untoward consequences, especially when the parents' exhaustion was exacerbated by insufficient sleep (Price 1991).

Clinicians in the private sector are usually insulated from both the medical and the social consequences of multiple births which occur in NHS hospitals. The concern that preoccupies IVF clinicians is elsewhere: to achieve an acceptable pregnancy rate. They are reluctant to risk a lower pregnancy rate by changing their practice. Moreover, they may be confronted with women and men who in the face of childlessness may well view a multiple pregnancy in a positive light. At the Universitaire Baudelocque in Paris, most couples (90 per cent) in the IVF programme were ready to take the risk of a triplet outcome to maximise their chances of a pregnancy (Contrepas 1989). Only 7 per cent of people attending the clinic expressed reservations about the possibility of multiple pregnancy and a few (3 per cent) declared themselves incapable of envisaging bringing up twins, quite apart from triplets.

In April 1988, the British IVF clinicians Fincham, Brinsden and Craft presented the results of a questionnaire survey of infertile couples attending the Humana Hospital, Wellington, London, an ILA-licensed centre in which they worked (Fincham *et al.* 1989). Although there are methodological difficulties with this survey, not least the low response rate (26.5 per cent), the results indicate some of the dilemmas faced. In response to the question 'How many babies would you ideally wish to deliver if fertility treatment was successful?', the majority of respondents (62 per cent) stated that they would wish to deliver twins, 29 per cent singletons, 5 per cent triplets. Just under 1 per cent stated a wish to deliver quadruplets or quintuplets. In an unpublished survey in New Jersey, Leiblum and her co-workers report that of four groups of women, three identified in terms of remedy sought, 'IVF, ovulation stimulation with human gonadotropins [HMG], donor insemination and female medical student', the 'IVF women' were 'the most receptive to having quadruplets or even quintuplets rather than having no biological children at all' (Leiblum *et al.* 1989).

The consultants I spoke to made it clear that in so far as there was any discussion with their patients about the number of eggs and embryos to be transferred, this was overlaid with a mutual concern about the prospect of pregnancy as an outcome of undergoing the procedure:

INTERVIEWER: Three [embryo transfers] would be your usual practice here?
FIRST CONSULTANT: Yes. We went down to two [embryo transfers] because we were concerned that we were getting too many multiples [multiple pregnancies]. The problem with IVF is the variability in the laboratory. When it's working well [you have] a high rate of pregnancy and a high rate of multiple pregnancy. When things are going not so well, the pregnancy rate falls and your multiples fall. And it's this balance between trying to get as many people pregnant as possible. I, personally, when I see couples, tell them this and try to steer them to two being put back, but there's three [embryos] going back at the present time.
SECOND CONSULTANT: I think the couples that I speak to – they'll say first do whatever to maximise my chances of getting pregnant. And they really don't see beyond that. Their goal is pregnancy. And if you talk to them about risks of miscarriage, risks of ectopics, risks of multiples, they don't want to know that. When what they want is to be *pregnant* and to have a child and they don't, the steps in between, don't seem to register.
INTERVIEWER: When you were putting two [embryos] back how were you presenting it to them?
SECOND CONSULTANT: Well, there were a number of couples who'd actually signed consent for three. Because they'd been to the clinic and they'd had one treatment cycle before we'd changed to two. And each of these couples was seen by one of the doctors and the situation was explained and they did agree. But, um, it's, to some extent, how you present it, isn't it?

A consultant in another IVF clinic expressed the view that most of the women and men attending his clinic 'couldn't comprehend what it was to have triplets. No doubt, I mean, they just saw this as a pregnancy. It's the only thing they see.' When he was asked how he made the decision between two and three embryos in general, he identified what he referred to as 'medical conditions' where he believed that a two-embryo transfer to the woman concerned would be indicated:

> There are certain medical conditions where twins are a disaster, never mind triplets. For example, a diabetic or a paraplegic. Or we had one woman who was on social security whose husband was blind . . . and she'd have to bring them up on supplementary wages and we would only put two back for her. She had a singleton, I'm pleased to say. And we had a paraplegic woman, who we only put two back. And so on. So I think there are medical conditions when you have every right to say to the patient that we advise you to have two put back.

INTERVIEWER: But your norm was three, was it?

CONSULTANT: The norm was three.

EGG DONATION

> Egg collection is an invasive procedure which can cause pain and discomfort to the woman concerned. It may also involve the use of superovulatory drugs.
>
> (Human Fertilisation and Embryology Authority Code of Practice: Explanation 1991: 9)

The pressure on the British government to regulate IVF practice arose not least because of the added complexity of donated eggs and sperm. For although the use of donor sperm creates no particular precedent when included in an IVF programme, this is not the case with egg donation. Egg donation is only possible with the techniques that were developed as part of IVF. Descriptions of pregnancies following the transfer of donated eggs did not appear in the *British Medical Journal* until 1983 and in *Nature* in 1984 (Trounson *et al.* 1983; Lutjen *et al.* 1984). Donor egg programmes have now been established worldwide and promoted recently as extending the prospect of childbearing to women aged over 40 (Navot *et al.* 1991).

For the Warnock Committee, the argument for egg donation was that this might provide some with 'the only chance of their having a child which the woman can carry to term, and which is the genetic child of her husband'. The Committee regarded egg donation as ethically acceptable 'where the donor has been properly counselled and is fully aware of the risks' (1984: 36). Reference is made in the Warnock Report to 'relatively minor surgical risks' to be faced by the donor which arise from the surgical intervention to collect the eggs. But these risks are not spelt out. Nor is there mention of the risks of ovarian hyper-stimulation syndrome, associated with the use of superovulatory drugs (Navot *et al.* 1988; Smith and Cooke 1991). Braude[7] has described this syndrome:

> [I]n this case the ovary can become very large, it can become the size of a rugby ball, it can cause extreme pain and you can get fluid in the abdomen and even fluid in the chest. Now all gynaecologists working in their field are aware of the syndrome which can occur to any patient having fertility treatment and are on the lookout for it. If it occurs as part of fertility treatment it can be understood that it is a natural consequence, or one of the side-effects one might expect. However, I think it'd be difficult to justify giving these high doses of drugs to women who are not on fertility treatment, merely for the purpose of getting eggs.

Recipients

To whom are donor programmes made available? Donor programmes were established explicitly to enable the prospect of a pregnancy for women previously diagnosed as irreversibly sterile: women with primary or secondary ovarian failure resulting from gonadal dysgenesis (Turner's syndrome), major deletions on one X chromosome, surgery, chemotherapy and/or radiotherapy or menopause. But the number of indications has been extended. Some clinicians now include women with normal menstrual cycles who have not responded to standard ovulation induction (Leeton *et al.* 1984); to women who have not become pregnant after repeated IVF or GIFT procedures; 'to infertile women over 40 years of age who are still menstruating' (Serhal and Craft 1989); and to women with 'familial genetic disorders that are difficult to diagnose by early prenatal diagnostic techniques (Huntingdon's chorea, fibrocystic disease of the pancreas etc.)' (Serhal 1990).

Who is to be excluded? With so many indications, there is no shortage of demand. Serr and his co-authors enthuse about the 'rejuvenation of the prematurely menopausal woman' now with some possibility of bearing a child. They then express their qualms about requests from women who 'by clinical standards' have 'passed the age of procreation':

> [P]roblems are beginning to arise as requests are submitted by

post-menopausal women in their late fifties for admission to the egg donation programme. They had been declared sterile during their childbearing years but had heard of the new technique through the media.

(1989: 32)

In Serhal and Craft's egg donation series, eleven of the twenty-nine women recipients who became pregnant at their clinic were over 42 years old. They concluded that 'fertility potential is high irrespective of the recipient's age' when eggs are donated by young women (Serhal and Craft 1989: 1187). Thus reproductive potential can be extended to women over 40 who have already entered the menopause. Sauer described four menopausal women, aged 40 to 44, who gave birth to live infants after egg donation (Sauer *et al.* 1990). Navot and his co-authors also enthusiastically promote egg donation for women who still have menstrual cycles to enable them to extend their reproductive potential (Navot *et al.* 1991). The HFEA Code of Practice now sets an age limit of 35 for egg donors. But it does not recommend an upper age limit for women who wish to be the recipients, regarding it as 'a matter for the centre and the clients to decide in the light of relevant information and counselling (if any)' (HFEA 1991). In March 1992, the private Lister Hospital in London announced that two 50-year-old women were about to give birth. Their partners were men aged 55 and 53. The pregnancies were established using eggs donated by younger women. The clinician involved was reported as saying: 'You have to draw the line somewhere, and we have drawn it at the age of natural menopause which is 49 or 50.' He added: 'You have to consider each case on its merits. It's not only a medical question but a moral and social problem.' He felt comfortable in making the decision. However, another IVF clinician is quoted as referring to the 'obvious problem' of 'very aged parents – when the child is 10, they'll be 60' (Crosbie 1992). The consequences of the bearing of a late *first* child on relationships and also the cultural effects of a growing awareness of the possibility of extended reproductive potential have yet to be explored.

Donors: known or anonymous

Eggs are chronically in short supply. So-called 'spare' eggs from women undergoing IVF or GIFT were the original source for donor programmes. But as the facility to cryo-preserve embryos became available, women and men claimed this opportunity to freeze their embryos for their own use at a later time.

The Warnock Committee advocated donor anonymity. However, they accepted that 'present practicalities' in egg collection and storage provided adequate grounds to make an exception 'where the egg was donated by a sister or close friend'. The rationale was not spelt out, but the Committee advocated that 'particularly careful counselling for all concerned would be necessary' (1984: 37).

Some clinicians in the United Kingdom argue strongly for kin, and particularly sisters, to be able to donate eggs for use by relatives in IVF and GIFT procedures. As one clinician put it:

> They're all situations where sisters would like to help sisters. You can understand that you might wish to have the same genetic background to an egg donated to you as you had of your parents. Why not? It doesn't necessarily mean to say it is going to be bad.[8]

Public attention was first drawn to this advocacy in 1986, when this same clinician agreed to relatives donating eggs to relatives (Fraser 1987; Veitch 1987). The clinician's rationale centred on facilitation and the value placed on genetic continuity: that women felt secure in the knowledge that donated eggs come from 'within the family', thus 'keeping it in the family gene pool'. A woman who received eggs donated by her sister described what this meant for her:

> With my sister's eggs we are continuing the family's bloodline – at least there is still that connection with my parents and grandparents.
> (Steven 1987:13)

Portrayed in terms of altruism ('a lovely gift'), the wider social implications of such donations remain unexplored. In publicly discussed 'known donor' situations, it is presumed that the transfer is between a relative or friend living in a separate household. By the nature of the relationship the donor is expected to be a continuing presence in the life of the recipient and her child. Perhaps the positive presentation of the idea of sisters giving eggs to sisters lies in the assumption that such relationships rest on a moral basis, or that the gift is unlikely to lead to future claims, material or otherwise, by the donor on the recipient or her child. In 1987, the Second Report of the VLA advised that egg donors should be, and should remain, anonymous. 'There are relationships within which the practice would be inadvisable,' the Authority considered (VLA 1987: 24). But its later version does not suggest actually forbidding the use of known donors:

> Egg donors should remain anonymous and for this reason donations

for clinical purposes from any known person including close relatives should be avoided.

(ILA 1990a)

Although it is expected that donations will be anonymous, the ILA information booklet *Egg Donation: Your Questions Answered*, available to all potential egg donors, mentions the possibility of exceptions 'for very rare cases' (ILA 1990a). At least one hospital ethical committee has defined such cases as 'being from an ethnic minority group'.[9]

In October 1986, members of a hospital ethical committee discovered that on one occasion a clinician had taken eggs from a niece to give to her aunt. Then, in December 1986, they learned about an even more controversial plan. The matron of the hospital had heard of it from one of her nurses and she reported it to the secretary of the ethical committee. On television, he recounted how he had intervened to prevent a transfer between a daughter and a mother in the hospital's IVF unit by informing the VLA of his concern.

> The nurse had admitted an 18-year-old girl, a Kenyan Asian and her 45-year-old mother and the intention was that eggs should be donated by the 18-year-old girl to her mother who had since remarried; the mother in fact had five children already and had remarried a 56 year old with three children of his own. . . . [Because of the particular circumstances] we were concerned as to whether there was any possibility that the 18-year-old daughter could have actually given a free and informed consent to the procedure. . . . So I rang some members of the Voluntary Licensing Authority at home that day and they concurred with my opinion and that of other people at the hospital that this was not a procedure that should be allowed to happen, and the medical director of the hospital saw [the consultant involved] the following day and asked him not to do it.[10]

The principle of anonymity is intended to eliminate the possibility of any relationship with the donor. In the case of sperm donation, the anonymity of donors is usually protected (Bolton *et al.* 1991; Haimes 1991). Nevertheless, the idea of donor anonymity remains a background controversy in clinical practice. There is uncertainty about the desirability of giving information to children conceived by sperm or egg donation (Braude *et al.* 1990; Bolton *et al.* 1991) and about people's practice. Several studies report that most parents of children who are the result of donor inseminations do not tell their children of this; that it is a well-kept secret (Berger *et al.* 1986). Such secrets function to articulate a boundary around those relationships which are to be regarded as parental, and as familial. Yet it has been argued that withholding information must create an atmosphere of deception (Department of Health and Social Security 1984; McWhinnie 1986; Glover *et al.* 1989). Secrets pose a challenge to those who are not privy to them. People who have been adopted have been deeply distressed by accidental disclosure of the facts about their adoption when these facts have previously been concealed from them. In a joint briefing paper, submitted in response to the Human Fertilisation and Embryology Bill, the British Agencies for Adoption and Fostering (BAAF) and the British Association of Social Workers asserted, 'Those receiving treatment services need to be aware, quite apart from the moral issues involved, of the impracticality of attempting to keep a secret of this nature' (BAAF 1990: 2).

Donors, for their part, may not regard their donation as a secret: at one clinic it seems that most egg donors (80 per cent) told friends, relatives or doctors (Power *et al.* 1990). Some donors have told their story to the press and on television. Section 31 of the Human Fertilisation and Embryology Act requires the HFEA to keep a register containing identifying information about people who are donors and of children born as a result of donation. The purpose is explicitly to enable the Authority to respond to requests from such children, once they reach the age of majority, as to whether or not they are related to their intended marriage partner. But there is tacit recognition that thereby they may ferret out secrets:

> The purpose of the register is to enable people over the age of 18 *who think they may have been born as a result of donation* to apply to the Authority for information about their origins. People who are contemplating marriage will also be able to apply to the Authority to find out whether there is a chance that they may be related to their intended spouse.
>
> (HFEA 1991; emphasis added)

Anonymous egg donors are likely to be women undergoing sterilisation procedures or women who volunteer following publicity. Women awaiting egg donation may also be encouraged to recruit donors for other women (Abdalla and Studd 1989). At least two clinics report that women who recruit donors will have priority in receiving eggs.

No secret is made about the shortage of donors, particularly from certain ethnic groups, and the need for the clinic to recruit donors if they wish to have a donor programme. Several clinics take eggs from women who are undergoing treatment on their assisted fertilisation programme: women in one clinic are asked to donate a maximum of six eggs if they produce more than twelve during their treatment cycle (Abdalla and Studd 1989; Power *et al.* 1990). The clinician concerned has no hesitation with this practice:

> Of course, using women who are about to be sterilised is best, but there are not enough of them. We need to get as many eggs as possible for infertile women.

> (McKie 1988)

Yet other clinics will not countenance donations either from women undergoing IVF or GIFT or sterilisation; some will accept one but not the other. At the same time, as more clinics establish egg donation programmes, the practice of using publicity to recruit women as donors is increasing (Abdalla and Studd 1989; Abdalla 1990).

Who donates and why? There are few data on the characteristics and motivations of donors. Nor is there information about the social conditions which might be conducive to donation. Women, it is generally reported in the clinical literature, donate for 'altruistic' reasons to enable other women to conceive (Leeton and Harman 1986; Power *et al.* 1990). But the clinical context itself may lend a reassurance to the idea of egg donation that is not present in sperm donation. Haimes (1991) has drawn attention to the cultural assumptions about gender which lead to egg and sperm donation being implicitly contrasted with one another, and particularly in relation to the motives which are ascribed to the donors. Her interviews with members of the Warnock Committee suggested that a sense of danger and the pathological lay behind discussions about sperm donation which was not evident in discussions about egg donation. Egg donation is necessarily contained within a clinical setting and is 'between' women. Consequently, Haimes suggests, such donations may be perceived as essentially asexual and supportive of rather than disruptive to traditional ideas about family. Concerns about the 'invasion of a third party' into the family are not raised in relation to egg donation as they are with sperm donation. Nevertheless, when egg donation was considered by itself, individual members of the Warnock Committee also expressed quite ambivalent views.

The same ambivalence has surfaced in practice as well as reflection. There are only a small number of studies on egg donation, which may account for the extrapolations some are prepared to make. For instance, the IVF clinician Schover and his co-workers compared a control group of women with women who had volunteered as egg donors in response to their recruiting publicity (Schover *et al.* 1990). Potential donors themselves reportedly referred to 'altruism', or, less frequently, financial gain, as their stated motivation. Yet Schover and his colleagues surmise: 'They may have a covert wish to expiate guilt over past sexual conduct or elective abortion or to compensate for the loss of a parent, sibling or child.' Just under half of these potential volunteers had a parent or sibling with 'a history of chemical dependency' and just over a sixth had 'a close family member with a major psychopathology'. Over a third reported a sexual trauma; about three-quarters had experienced 'at least one reproductive trauma'; and the majority had at least one family disruption (Schover *et al.* 1990). All the potential egg donors in Schover's study had also been screened by the clinic. This included the completion of a very time-consuming per-sonality profile (the Minnesota Multiphasic Personality Inventory). As a consequence, less than a fifth of the volunteers were in fact accepted 'without reservation as donors. Yet other volunteers about whom they had reservations were also accepted on the programme on the grounds that the clinic would otherwise have difficulty in matching donors with potential recipients.

Clinicians may feel concerned about the motivations of certain of their donors. Some of those I interviewed expressed anxiety. One consultant reported to me: 'We had one crank, who I think was trying to test us out, you know. . . . We knew she was a bit strange. But we let her slip through.' Schover and his co-workers seemingly accept the fact that donors may be attempting restitution for previous psychological loss: they also find it plausible that donating oocytes is a 'healthy way for some women to deal with feelings about past traumatic experiences'. However tentatively such ideas are put forward, comfortable ideas about an unexplored sense of altruism in relation to egg donation have been disturbed.

CONCLUSION: WHAT KIND OF FACILITATION?

The advent of IVF was, without doubt, a landmark in reproductive medi-cine. Lesley Brown's pregnancy and the birth of her daughter Louise in 1978 following IVF and the transfer of a single cleaving embryo to her uterus were the sought-after proof that clinicians could bypass a woman's blocked or damaged fallopian tubes and give her the hope of a pregnancy. However, professional concerns have mounted not only as a consequence of the rise in numbers of multiple pregnancies of three or more but also as the indications for IVF are extended far beyond the bypassing of blocked fallopian tubes.

The use of donated gametes has revived opinions which were strongly voiced in relation to donor insemination earlier this century (Archbishop of Canterbury's Commission 1948; Home Office and Scottish Home

Department 1960). The setting up of egg donation programmes and sur-rogacy 'services' has also triggered anxieties about just who is responsible for what in this field of medicine, especially when the promotional lan-guage is of remedy and, increasingly, of substitution. Literally, one per-son's gametes may be substituted for those of another. Metaphorically speaking, the whole search for alternative routes to pregnancy may be regarded as a matter of finding substitutes for impaired organs and capaci-ties. Who is to set the standards for screening, evaluation, counselling and informed consent? In the public debates anticipating the Human Fertilisa-tion and Embryology Act, there was widespread support for the idea that people seeking clinical services to alleviate infertility should be enabled to make more informed decisions and to envisage and take responsibility for the possible consequences.

In many countries, such concerns have pushed infertility services high up on public policy agendas. But to what effect? Change is anticipated: there is regulation and review. Yet within the policy arena in the United Kingdom, preconceived ideas about the standing of medical decisions in clinical practice remain highly influential and encourage certain policy conclusions.

This is a particular kind of facilitation. Institutional pressures protect the established status of clinical judgement, which thus becomes used to control the discourse about risk. Medical practitioners are accustomed both to being authoritative in decision-making and to having autonomous control of their activities. In the absence of any appraisal of the possible social implications or the complexity of the relationships involved, decisions usually have to be made by clinicians on pragmatic grounds. This involves decisions about the criteria which must be met before treat-ment services are provided, or a potential donor or surrogate recruited. Clinicians who claim that they legitimately have discretion, that such mat-ters call for their professional judgement, receive influential endorsement (Dunstan 1989). Some also act, in effect, as 'guarantors' in IVF surrogacy arrangements. There are also clinicians who publicly promote personal views about anonymity and secrecy in relation to gamete donation. Yet other clinicians are uneasy: they perceive the extent to which they have been vested with an authority of a moral kind where the facilitation of pregnancy is concerned.

Facilitation of pregnancy is already in the public domain when it takes place with the intervention of clinicians. The clinical presence itself inevit-ably influences views about the options available. When, in their quest for a pregnancy, women and men seek medical assistance, clinicians find themselves mediating not just the technical facilities or the information available but mediating between parties to relationships of various kinds.

There is a pressing need to explore both the ways in which notions such as risk are perceived and how clinical authority and the institution of medicine variously reinforce or create the ways in which they make their choices. And how the doubts and concerns that surface in the course of clinical practice are also to be heard. Acts of assistance can be undermined by untoward consequences.

NOTES

1 Jonathan Glover, 'Antenna', BBC, 24 October 1987.
2 Van Noord-Zaadstra and his co-workers in the Netherlands pinpointed 31 as the age at which the decline in fecundity begins and after which the chance of having a healthy baby decreases (van Noord-Zaadstra *et al.* 1991). Women older than 31 take longer to become pregnant than younger women; after 45 pregnancy becomes very unlikely. Endometrial vasculature, uterine blood supply and the quality of eggs have been implicated in this decline in fertility (Schwartz *et al.* 1982; Stein 1985; Gosden 1985; Medical Research International Society for Assisted Reproductive Technology 1991; Navot *et al.* 1991; van Noord-Zaadstra *et al.* 1991).
3 Quoted in a memorandum from Nicola Gooch, London Weekend Television, about 'The London Programme', 12 September 1990.
4 As elsewhere in this chapter, clinicians' comments are taken from taped transcriptions of interviews.
5 The VLA was a voluntary, non-statutory body. It had no 'teeth' and relied on peer group pressure. Its only sanction was the stigma of the withdrawal of its licence. It became the ILA in order to draw attention to its provisional status.
6 Also the Medical Research Council (MRC) Working Party on Children Conceived by In Vitro Fertilisation reported that up to the end of 1987, 23 per cent of deliveries following assisted conception by IVF or GIFT had resulted in a multiple birth of twins or more, compared with about 1 per cent for natural conception (MRC 1990). There is the additional risk factor of a higher than expected frequency of identical (monozygotic) twins, not only after the induction of ovulation with drugs but also after IVF and GIFT (Edwards *et al.* 1986; Derom *et al.* 1987; Price 1989). Thus there are reports of three eggs or embryos being transferred in a GIFT or IVF procedure and the outcome being a quadruplet pregnancy.
7 Peter Braude, 'The First Fourteen Days' (television transcript, p. 12), 'Horizon', BBC, 26 February 1990.
8 Ian Craft, 'Antenna', BBC, 24 October 1987.
9 'Our Ethical Committee has defined such circumstances as being from an ethnic minority group,' The Lister Hospital 'Ovum Donation' information sheets, n.d.
10 Richard Nicholson, 'Antenna', BBC, 24 October 1987.

Afterword for Chapter 1

'Solutions for Life and Growth'? Collaborative conceptions in reproductive medicine

Frances Price

The image that dominates a recent advertisement in the scientific journal *Human Reproduction* shows exultant Berliners perched atop the wall that once partitioned East from West.[1] The caption reads: 'A change of culture can be radical to an adult. Imagine the impact on an embryo.' The advertiser, the multi-national biomedical company Medi-Cult, trades in 'Solutions for Life and Growth'. On sale is a solution in a bottle: 'culture media' for keeping human embryos alive in the laboratory.[2]

The company claims a breakthrough in embryo culture, a new-and-improved culture that will assist embryos to achieve 'optimal growth conditions with minimal risk of metabolic shock'. The image promises more, as it celebrates the symbolic moment of political change and economic transformation, when free trade supplanted state socialism. Buy a culture, and buy into a culture – the market is promoted as the source of progress in the field of reproductive medicine and political economy alike.

The marriage of medicine and the market, however, creates a political alliance that is particularly potent when the practices involved bring new persons into being. Bolstered by the unique authority of the institution of medicine and the established status of clinical judgement, clinicians are well placed to shape the context in which they practice (Kerr *et al.* 1997). Deploying the vocabulary of supply and demand combined with a humanitarian rhetoric, they can successfully promote the development and maintenance of 'efficient clinical services' in both public and private domains, influencing government policy, industrial investment and media coverage. Moreover, clinicians increasingly act as key mediators of scientific innovation in human genetics and reproduction, conveying new developments from the laboratory into the clinic (Price 1996). These influences are of special concern in reproductive medicine, not least because the focus for both clinician and patient is the facilitation of a pregnancy, contextualised within a medical frame centred on the individualised 'case'

– a prioritisation that obscures a wider context in terms of connection and relationship between persons.

Five years on from the publication of the first edition of *Technologies of Procreation*, clinical teams working to produce and culture embryos have fostered continuing confidence that there can be solutions to intractable infertility. As demands for such services escalate, the notion of substituting gametes in the making of embryos has become widespread. Most recently, the idea of substitution has become allied with the prospect of 'copying'. The prospect of 'reproductive cloning' has emerged as another novel technique promising not only 'biological' connection but also genetic predictability.

During the 1990s, the substitution of gametes has become available as a standard procedure. In particular, clinical services designed to establish pregnancies using eggs acquired from other women have become established as one of the most successful forms of infertility treatment. However, the acquisition of human eggs for substitution remains problematic.[3]

In Britain, since the origins of the practice in the mid-1980s, only eggs 'donated' by women without financial inducement have been made available for transfer to other women. Increasingly, however, market terminology dominates policy discussions. Some clinicians argue on pragmatic grounds that egg 'providers' should be paid to meet a marked shortage of donated gametes which has not been met by recruitment campaigns organised by clinics. As one British infertility specialist, Ian Craft, argues:

> I favour egg donation without financial reward, but the demand for eggs far outstrips the supply from women who donate for altruistic reasons. . . . My preference is probably unrealistic in today's world, where money determines health care. Our prime concern is to provide an efficient clinical service.
>
> (Craft 1997: 1400)

In the United States, a trade in human eggs is now entrenched in the repertoire of services provided by private fertility clinics operating in an unregulated market place. This trade, however, is the most heavily criticised aspect of reproductive technology. Mark Sauer, a clinician foremost in the field in the US, remarks:

> Today in the USA, groups openly advertise and aggressively solicit young women to participate. A decade ago, the idea of unmarried, nulliparous women, typically still in school, undergoing an invasive procedure . . . was unthinkable [given the risks involved]. So what's

different today? Labelling the practice standard or conventional seems to have justified it . . . issues of supply and demand have become paramount. . . . 10 years ago, donors received $250 per cycle, today, $2,500 is not uncommon.

(Sauer 1996: 1149)

When money is the inducement for a woman to provide her eggs for the use of another woman, the medical management of the risks associated with the hormonal treatment and egg retrieval operation presents special difficulties. Mark Sauer points to 'an inherent moral ambiguity in a practice of medicine that simultaneously places young women at risk of infertility while treating the childlessness of other women' (Sauer 1997).

Despite such concerns, the idea that human gametes provided for others should come within the embrace of the market in the UK has gained ground, in the wake of sustained media interest in 'waiting lists' for eggs.[4] Another vocabulary is in play, however. 'There is a strong social ethos in Britain of voluntary unpaid donation, such as blood and tissue donation,' Martin Johnson, a leading research embryologist at the University of Cambridge, argues (Johnson 1997: 1402). He is also a member of the regulatory body for IVF and embryo research, the Human Fertilisation and Embryology Authority. The HFEA, he states, is concerned 'not to erode in any way the culture of voluntary unpaid donation that currently exists for egg donation. Rather, it wishes to strengthen and develop this culture.'[5] He writes of his concern that 'to pay donors might lead them to be marginalised by both the clinics and recipients as being simply a means to an end'.

In Britain, recent research suggests that women who currently donate would not donate for payment (Abdalla 1996; Price 1998). Here, egg donation has been conceptualised in terms of altruism and expressed as cultural performance: recruitment advertisements urge women to 'Give the gift of life', or ask, 'Are you the kind of woman who could make another woman pregnant?' My current research demonstrates that women who volunteer to give their eggs to another woman are made to feel special, with far-reaching consequences for their identity and the social support available to them: in so far as they are perceived to be acting benevolently, donors elicit help and goodwill from others.[6] As one egg donor remarked to me:

They all thought I was wonderful at the GP's surgery [where she went for her hormone injections to induce multiple ovulation]. They made me feel as though I was quite unusual. They made me feel quite special, in fact.[7]

In 1996, the HFEA announced its intention to phase out all payments for human gametes, although it authorised the continuation of existing practice during a 'transitional period'. The HFEA's announcement of intent is in effect a step back from payment in favour of 'unisex altruism' for both sperm and egg donors (Dickenson 1997). The announcement created a furore among many clinicians, however, leading the HFEA to circulate a public consultation document, *Consultation on the Implementation of Withdrawal of Payment to Donors* (HFEA, February 1998, which at the time of writing is still on-going).

Gamete donation opens up novel issues in relation to donors, recipients and any children born of the donation (Price 1997). Unfamiliar dimensions of risk and uncertainty arise, as do questions of connection, accountability and responsibility. Yet these issues go largely unexamined – not least because gametes are transferred between individuals as part of an increasingly familiar HFEA-licensed 'treatment service'. Here, medical mediation typically maintains a separation between donor and recipient: their relationship within the clinic has come to be defined predominantly in therapeutic terms, with the donor doing the 'work' of a patient despite not being perceived as one.[8] Furthermore, the medical framing of these services acts to obscure the complex contexts in which, beyond the clinic, outcomes are experienced, and may or may not elicit social support. Moreover, a relationship exists between even an anonymous donor and recipient as each configure the other (Price 1995).

At the same time as it promotes the prospect of solutions for 'intractable infertility', whether female or male, the medical profession encourages the demand for innovative technologies, which often involve the substitution of one element of a body for another. This is nowhere more clear than in the celebration, by some clinicians, of the 'promise' of cloning humans – the creation of infants that are potentially genetically identical copies of an adult, using the technique of 'nuclear replacement': the substitution of one genome for another. The birth of just one lamb, Dolly – produced using DNA extracted from an adult ewe's udder cell by scientists at Roslin Institute near Edinburgh – has brought the possible cloning of humans to the fore (Wilmut *et al.* 1997). Some infertility specialists anticipate 'using cloning methods to help couples have babies of their own – even, perhaps, babies who were actual clones' (Kolata 1997).

Robert Winston, a prominent British infertility clinician, welcomes 'the promise of cloning for human medicine' (Winston 1997: 913). In his view, cloning should 'not be seen as a moral threat but rather as an exciting challenge'; it offers, for example, a potential solution for a man who exhibits 'total germ cell failure', and so cannot produce even immature sperm cells. A male infant could in theory be produced from his DNA, through 'nuclear transfer'.

Who would be the boy's parents? Winston does not refer to a 'father'. He does, however, introduce 'the mother'. By providing a denucleated egg to house the infertile man's genetic material, a woman 'would contribute important constituents' to the man's clone. Her contribution would be partly genetic: her egg cytoplasm would contribute a small number of 'mitochondrial' genes.[9] Were she also to gestate and give birth, she would provide 'intra-uterine influences' as well. Were she to look after the child, she would additionally provide 'subsequent nurture'.

For Winston, a sufficient account of the relational consequences of cloning is one that thus apportions the relative contributions attributable to 'genes' or 'environment': 'we are a product of our nurture as much as our genetic nature,' he asserts (Winston 1997: 914). Yet the neglected issue here is not the reality of biological connection, nor the importance of nurture, but how the cloning of humans is to be imagined, debated and made culturally meaningful. In Winston's account, the claims between persons, the ensuing relationships, and the social context in which these relations gain support – all are tacitly presumed to be unproblematic.

How has this come to pass? Medical authority may confer an image of reassuring competence whilst endorsing and structuring particular kinds of options and interventions. Certain considerations have been brought to the fore to the exclusion of others, especially when the promotional language is of remedy and increasingly of substitution. Embedded in medical practice, substitution in a range of contexts acquires a legitimacy that readily accrues to practices within the clinical remit.

Who is responsible for what in this field of medically managed solutions, in which the goal is to facilitate pregnancies for an increasingly wide spectrum of would-be parents? How is it possible to think about the implications of new reproductive technologies for relationships between persons and generations? As new-and-improved solutions for embryo culture continue to be developed and marketed, *Technologies of Procreation* ventures to open to scrutiny the culture of solutions that now dominates practice in this field of medicine and which has largely set the agenda for public debate.

NOTES

1 Advertisement in *Human Reproduction*, 12 (4), April 1997.
2 Pre-implantation embryos normally develop within the protective environment of the female reproductive tract. Research embryologists continue to

attempt to improve culture media capable of supporting embryonic development. For a discussion of some of the issues at the forefront of the quest for improved culture media, see B.D. Bavister (1995) 'Culture of preimplantation embryos: facts and artifacts', *Human Reproduction Update 1995*, 1 (2), 91–148; M.H. Johnson and M.H. Nars-Esfahani (1994) 'Radical solutions and cultural problems: could free oxygen radicals be responsible for the impaired development of pre-implantation mammalian embryos in vitro?' *BioEssays*, 16: 31–8.

3 Changing clinical practice has acted to increase demand, as egg donation has been expanded to include as recipients post-menopausal women, ovulating women classified as 'IVF failures', and women who have repeatedly miscarried.

4 Commercialisation is proffered as necessary to the reliable provision of a medical treatment for which there is popular demand, as an advertisement placed in the London *Times* in 1994 (7 August) underlines. Headed 'Donor Egg. Immediate Availability, No Waiting List,' the advertisement announced that the Genetics and IVF Institute of Fairfax, Virginia, has 'a large selection of donors available now for patients requiring donor eggs'. By contrast, women seeking egg donation in Britain may spend some two years on a waiting list in the private sector of medicine and far longer on National Health Service waiting lists.

5 The Human Fertilisation and Embryology Act 1990 specified that 'no money or other benefit shall be given or received in respect to any supply of gametes or embryos unless authorised by Directions'. However, to avoid disruption to service provision that immediate withdrawal of any form of payment would cause, the HFEA advised fertility clinics that they could continue to pay donors. In current practice, the HFEA allows clinics that were paying (*de facto* sperm) donors £15 plus reasonable expenses before 1 August 1991 to continue to do so (HFEA, 'Giving and receiving money or other benefits in respect of any supply of gametes or embryos', General Directions, D. 1996/1, Manual for Centres, Version 2.2, March 1996). Egg donors currently are offered travel and (sometimes) childcare expenses and can also receive sterilisation or fertility treatment in return for donating gametes. The desire to bring egg donation in line with sperm donation has fuelled the campaign to introduce payments. The perceived need for financial inducements for sperm donation arose in the 1950s in a climate that associated stigma and secrecy with sperm donation, but this has not been the history of egg donation. See K. Daniels, and E. Haimes, (eds) (1998) *Donor Insemination: International Social Science Perspectives*, Cambridge: Cambridge University Press.

6 My research on egg donation combined ethnographic fieldwork in clinics with in-depth interviews with women in Britain who have been, or are about to become, donors or recipients of human eggs. Little is known about how or why women decide to give or receive eggs, or how egg donation impinges upon ideas about identity and kinship as new social and legal relationships are forged between those 'collaborating' in such medically mediated conceptions. The study was funded by grants from the Nuffield Foundation and from the Isaac Newton Trust, University of Cambridge.

7 From transcript of interview with egg donor, 'Collaborative Conceptions' project, see note above.

8 For example, a study by Roberta Lessor of egg donation between sisters in a large university IVF centre in the United States has documented the unprecedented difficulties that arise. See R. Lessor (1993) 'All in the family: social processes in ovarian egg donation between sisters', *Sociology of Health and Illness*, 15: 393–413.

9 Hypothetically, cloning a man must involve one or more women, as egg donor and surrogate mother. The man's DNA must first be placed in an egg cell that has had its nucleus removed; the egg retains some DNA in the form of genes within the mitochondria, energy-producing organelles that each embryo inherits via the egg. The resulting embryo must then be transferred to a woman's womb to develop to term. In Britain, the legal mother is the woman who gives birth.

2 Explicit connections
Ethnographic enquiry in north-west England

Jeanette Edwards

Forms of reproductive assistance are and will continue to be a focus of concern in many spheres of contemporary life. While the medical and legal professions ponder the practical and ethical conundrums arising alongside – if nor a step behind – scientific developments in reproductive medicine, feminist observers, among others, ask questions about who benefits from reproductive technology. At the same time, those who require fertility services are concerned with the need for increased and equal access to appropriate and adequate treatment. To take an anthropological approach to the impact of new reproductive technology (NRT) is to take an interest in perspectives: the fact that forms of reproductive assistance have become a focus of concern in many spheres of contemporary life becomes an issue in itself. Such an anthropological approach would not only explore the same phenomenon from different viewpoints, including those of different interest groups, it would also look to locate those perspectives in a wider cultural context. Ideas about 'new reproductive technology' are to be understood in the context of other ideas which inform the viewpoint people take, and are informed by it. The premise of the present chapter is that these will include notions about relatedness and reproducing persons which go beyond the immediate issues of fertility and conception.

Our project as a whole both tries to make some of these perspectives evident and offers a perspective itself. We have seen (Chapter 1) how, at IVF centres across the country, clinicians in the context of daily interactions with their clients have to make decisions about who should be eligible for their services and what type of assistance is appropriate. Members of Parliament, for their part, must debate a rather different range of issues in the context of formulating legislative guidelines (see Chapter 4). If these perspectives are given by the arena of debate, our studies constituted other arenas and elicited further perspectives. In a town in the north-west of England ('Alltown'), people who have no vested interest in NRTs were invited to discuss and analyse what they perceive to be the implications of different techniques of assisted conception. This is the basis of the material considered here. The chapter that follows (Chapter 3) focuses on households in London, where married couples negotiate the views they present to the researcher in the context of their relationship and what they understand of each other's wider views and preoccupations. And if such perspectives can be seen to draw on pre-existing (cultural) assumptions, the same is true of the project itself. Academia offers a cultural context of sorts. Here anthropologists debate meanings of kinship and the significance – or not – to diverse cultures of the 'biological facts of life'.

Across these different contexts, people are drawing upon common, culturally specific, understandings of kinship. Thus, while each perspective can be treated as analytically distinct, each is also composed of a myriad of ideas and viewpoints on certain common issues that thereby occur and recur in different forms. It is from this further perspective that they constitute the kinship system which for present purposes may be called English (see also Strathern 1992a: 23).

THE CONTEXT: PRACTICE AND PREMISE

I see our project as concerned with the way in which ideas about kinship, in the light of technological developments in assisted conception, can be retrieved and analysed. This is a question not only relevant to method but one that also goes to the heart of theoretical underpinnings of social anthropology. The assumptions with which the project began cannot be dissociated from the practice which ensued. If we start with the premise that human reproduction not only creates new human beings but also kin relations, we are led to consider just how assisting conception technologically will implicate kinship. From this perspective, the topic of NRT acts as an ethnographic window through which kinship ideas and assumptions can be discerned. It is no surprise perhaps that anthropologists are not alone in this endeavour. The idea of technologically assisted conception makes a problematic out of the processes of human reproduction. In such a context, it is not only anthropologists who are compelled to explore the ways in which people are related.

The topic of new reproductive technology raised with some of the residents of Alltown elicited two dominant views which, at first glance, appear irreconcilable. The first is that infertile couples suffer a great deal of heartache and pain and should therefore be helped by whatever means are available. The second is that interference in the natural processes of reproduction is dangerous and certain possibilities for assisting conception are inappropriate and unacceptable for the 'growing of babies'. These two responses do not preclude each other and people do not adhere to one or other point of view. Yet the apparent opposition does not necessarily imply a fickleness or contradiction on the part of those presenting then. Indeed, a similar point is made in a different arena in Chapter 4. Alltown people present a diversity of perspectives among themselves – that they appear contradictory is partly a function of their juxtaposition in this analysis.

There might be a temptation to refer to fieldwork in the 'community' as being concerned with a popular understanding of NRT, or to expect an anthropological approach to uncover and highlight 'public opinion'. This is not my aim. Data collected in the context of my discussions with Alltown people will not be distilled into a common denominator which represents 'an opinion'; rather, my aim is to reflect how they contextualise ideas. In this account, I intend to preserve the way in which people formulate their views and the way in which they shift their individual perspectives according to the problem they are addressing.

I had previously conducted twelve months residential fieldwork in Alltown and returned in November 1990 (this time as a commuter) with the topics of kinship and the new reproductive technologies in mind. I was able to build on a prior knowledge of, and a familiarity with, the town and many of its residents, which thus forms the context of the present exercise. Before I explore ways in which Alltown people discussed techniques and implications of assisted conception with me, a brief and necessarily selective picture of the locality is necessary.

Alltown is in the north of England, the last in a ribbon development of towns and villages along a valley floor. It grew with the development of the textile industry in the region and by the middle of the nineteenth century was a busy and industrious milltown, attracting working-class families and individuals from different rural areas of England and Ireland. The terraced and back-to-back houses, built for the millworks and left empty when the cotton mills closed and workers moved elsewhere in search of employment, were either flattened during the slum clearance programmes of the 1950s and 1960s or renovated and sold as 'desirable cottages' during the 1980s. Over the past two decades, working-class immigrants in search of work have been replaced by middle-class immigrants in search of 'the country'. A small but steady influx of households whose members are either retired or commute to work have moved to Alltown, mainly from the nearby urban conurbation. This most recent wave of 'incomers'[1] appears to have halted the decline in population which at present stands at about 15,000 people. Most of the mills have since been demolished and the few that remain have been partially converted into shoe factories ('slipper works') or split into smaller industrial units. Short-time, redundancy and low pay are as much a feature of the manufacturing industry of the late twentieth century (particularly acute at present) as they were in the cotton mills of the late nineteenth century.

Certain patronyms are thought to be 'proper' Alltown names; others are associated with 'families' whose 'roots' are said to be in Ireland. Most present-day inhabitants who describe themselves as Alltown 'born and bred' trace their origins to immigrant labourers who arrived in the town during the second half of the nineteenth century. While many of the people I spoke to would claim such origins, others consider themselves and are considered to be 'incomers', either recent or well-established. This chapter draws on conversations with thirty-four Alltown residents between the ages of 21 and 90. I raised the topic of reproductive technology with some residents on more than one occasion; I was able to take notes during the majority of conversations and eight, including those with individuals as well as those between friends and between a group of women, were tape-recorded.

The information on which my account is based was given to me by people who themselves were not directly involved in NRTs; they were not undergoing treatments for infertility. There are two points to draw from this statement. The first is that my subjects were not patients. My questioning was directed at residents of a particular locality who, politeness notwithstanding, could refuse to talk to me. Access to them was negotiated at a personal level (rather than, say, a particular organisation of which they were clients). There was neither a vested interest nor, I think, a perceived obligation on their part to talk to me – other, that is, than the impelling but ordinary social obligations we all feel to be necessary within relationships. The second point is that although the people with whom I have spoken were not involved in NRTs, they were actively involved in a network of kinsfolk – either present or absent; they 'do' kinship.

In what follows, I will make a distinction between kin 'relationships' which I use to describe affective ties between kin, and kin 'relatedness' which I use to represent the abstract connections between those who are perceived as kin, the connections which in a sense do nothing but represent much. This distinction corresponds to a certain extent with Schneider's contrast between 'relationships as natural substance and relationship as code for conduct' (1980: 29). I wish, however, to extend the concept of relatedness beyond the presence of natural substance and use it to include notions of connectedness with or without a genetic link. Furthermore, kin relationships may *include* a code for conduct but such a code is not an imperative, and relationships take a variety of forms (see also Finch 1989: 241).

During 1990, I sought out those with whom I had maintained contact and resumed contact with other residents I had worked with when living in the town. My initial explorations into the way they perceive implications of assisted conception were thus carried out with people I met and have got to know since 1987/88. Any observations I make, therefore, are inevitably drawn from a wider and more diffuse understanding than that gained through interviews or conversations on the specific topic of NRTs. My interpretation is grounded in a familiarity with Alltown gained over time, not only through residential fieldwork and writing but also through successive visits and enduring ties with some residents. In turn, the people with whom I spoke defined the project and what was required themselves, not only from my descriptions of it but also from what they understood as the kind of 'work' I do, and from what they perceived I already knew about the town and its residents.

Some Alltown women became interested in the topic of research beyond our discussions and collected and presented me with clippings from newspapers or women's magazines. On more than one occasion, I was called at home and told of items that had been on the television or of forthcoming programmes that might interest me. People referred me to acquaintances whom they thought I might find interesting; often I was 'passed on' to people who it was perceived could provide an opposing or contrasting point of view, maybe because they were younger, or childless, or grandparents, or thought to be 'more traditional', or 'more liberal'. One woman advised that she was not a 'good person' for me to speak to as having had only one child she was obviously not 'very fertile'.

My aim is to present ideas about NRT both in the terms that Alltown people use and in a manner that indicates the way in which certain ideas lead on to other ideas. Of interest here are the analogies people draw upon in order to make sense of phenomena of which they have no direct experience but which nevertheless concern them profoundly. I make no apologies, therefore, in quoting extensively from Alltown. And while agreeing with Schneider (1980: 124) that these quotations serve to illustrate rather than prove an argument, I have to disagree with his point that such additions are a form of cheating. Like Alltown anecdotes, the examples I select might make proof to the contrary difficult, but what they do render visible is my understanding. I use them, then, to exemplify the way in which in Alltown ideas trigger other ideas. As I have already indicated, when thinking about possibilities presented through technological development in reproduction, people continually make analogies with what they already know; they model new possibilities on old facts. In so doing, they make explicit those 'facts', and render visible to themselves what used to be taken for granted.

MAKING EXPLICIT: KINSHIP LINKS

> In Marjory Proops' column this young man had an affair many years
> back with an older woman, a family friend. Then she came to be expect-
> ing this baby and she said it was his. Then he didn't want to know, so
> she said: 'Perhaps it's my husband's anyway.' So it's gone on now and
> his *own* son's grown up and they've got together, and they've got a very
> close relationship and he's asking [Marjory Proops] whether it should
> all come out or not.

One morning, during the half-term school holidays, I sat with a tape
recorder at Paula Seddon's kitchen table. Paula is in her mid-thirties with
four children between the ages of 5 and 17. In the front room a bevy of
young children were being kept amused by my son and one of Paula's sons
(12 and 14 years old respectively); children were constantly 'escaping' into
the kitchen, interceding with requests of their own. The presence of the
children acted as an apt reminder of reproductive conundrums. Mary
Greenwood, in her late fifties with two adult sons and four grandchildren,
joined us and told us a story, part of which I quote above. She had read the
letter that week in a magazine and told me that at the time it had reminded
her of me and what I was 'working' on now.

Why should Mary be reminded of new reproductive technology in the
age-old subject of infidelity and its attendant secrets? But then the question
asked of Marjory Proops was not, of course, about infidelity, but about
incest: should the young couple be allowed to form an intimate relationship not knowing that they are, in fact, related? One man I asked about
NRT in general responded immediately that it all sounded 'a bit incestuous' to him. A preoccupation which comes up again and again in Alltown
considerations of NRT is that children born through procedures of assisted
conception, unaware that they are genetically related, will 'meet up and
marry'.

Most of the Alltown people with whom I spoke weighed up the advantages and disadvantages of using sperm and eggs from anonymous and
known donors. One the one hand, it was argued, it was probably better to
'keep it in the family', while on the other using anonymous gametes would
prevent donors from 'interfering'. If the origin of gametes is unknown and
distant, then the disadvantage is that children born through such intervention will be unable to trace their 'roots' or know their genetic 'make-up'.
Gamete material which is known and close in its origin is conceptualised in
terms of incest. These two notions are juxtaposed in a common prediction
that artificial insemination by anonymous donor is bound to result, acci-
dentally but inexorably, in future incestuous relationships. The danger is

represented in the prediction that siblings, unaware of their relatedness, will meet up in the future and reproduce; further evidence is added to the inevitability of this scenario with the adage 'like attracts like'.

The idea of unknown genetic origins prompts people to think about kinship. And when kinship is part of the equation, incest is raised as a boundary or a limit which ought not to be traversed. I am concerned here with the symbolic import of incest[2] (cf. La Fontaine 1988; Bell 1991), and would argue that incest acts as a powerful conceptual brake to some of the possibilities presented through NRT. It represents a conceptual limit to ways of thinking about how persons and relationships should be reproduced. (Later, we shall see how the idea of 'cloning' acts as a similar conceptual limit to other possibilities presented in reproductive medicine.) But what is here presented as a chain of consequences for genetic connection is only part of a wider contextualisation of such concerns in relations based on kinship. When people draw on what they already know to order and make sense of the ramifications of NRT, they frequently turn to analogies with the kinds of problems that arise in complex family relationships, such as those formed through divorce and adoption. Complexity is apparent in the very combination of elements that contribute to the fact of relationship itself.

I asked one young woman what she meant by the 'bloodline', an expression she had used when exploring whom she would define as family. She explained: 'It's a line through which genetic characteristics are passed down.' Relatedness is created through blood or marriage. 'Real' relatives are those perceived to be connected by shared substance and for this purpose blood and genes appear to be intertwined. At the same time, certain characteristics of children are said to develop through their experiences in the womb. Hence, another young woman described how her youngest daughter is, as a baby, more robust and alert than were her three sons at a similar age. She explained that the baby had become accustomed to her voice:

> Raise my voice and she doesn't flinch; she was bashed about more in the womb[3] – so she's tougher.

Bringing these ideas to bear on the issue of surrogacy, a different woman with two adult children spoke of the 'influences' that a baby born of a surrogate mother will have received before birth:

> And what influences does it . . . the child [have] off its mother, through the umbilical cord. It's not receiving those influences from the person who is actually going to be its legal mother at the end of the process.

In talking hypothetically about surrogacy, people often symbolised the relationship between the carrying woman and child through a notion of shared substance mediated by the placenta; this connection requires neither a genetic link nor that the carrying woman assume a maternal role after the birth of the child. In other contexts, parents may be defined with reference to being 'real', so, for example, adoptive or step parents are sometimes said to act more like parents than the 'real' parents.[4] Non-genetic surrogacy presents the alternatives that the 'real' mother may be the person who gives birth to the child (particularly if viewed from the perspective of the surrogate mother) or the 'real' mother could be the provider of the egg (especially if viewed from the perspective of commissioning parents).

The idea of carrying a baby for another gives people pause for thought.[5] Many Alltown people with whom I spoke were disturbed by what they saw as the inevitable difficulty in 'giving up' a baby one had given birth to. One woman, while weighing up the possibility of donating an egg, compared egg donation with gestational surrogacy. She went on to think about whether she could act as a non-genetic surrogate:

> Would you say that's really my child – there's no bond to an egg? [I] couldn't surrogate – you'd never forget that the child came out of your body.

In a tape-recorded conversation with Keith and Lucy Davis in an Alltown pub,[6] I asked Keith first of all about his own family relationships and his role as a father. He talked at length about his relationship with his brothers and his two sons, and noted that his sisters were 'closer' to his mother and his sons 'closer' to his wife than he. I went on to ask him whether the ideas about obligations and expectations of help and assistance between family members, which he had been talking about, extended to help when members could not have children. He replied, 'there are medical reasons for not keeping it in the family, but if you couldn't [nodding to Lucy], I couldn't see why [my brother] couldn't be donor'. Keith went on to talk about IVF by donor which led him to raise the topic of surrogacy. It is evident from the ensuing conversation that, for him, surrogacy arrangements are more problematic than the donation of eggs and sperm. He made an analogy between the baby in a surrogate arrangement and eggs and sperm being donated and said he 'cannot visualise how anybody carrying a baby would want to part with it', whereas eggs and sperm are 'just matter . . . an egg is flushed away once a month and sperm is just body fluid'.

Another Alltown man, Alan Thomas, made a similar comparison, arguing that the baby 'belongs' to the woman who carries it and that surrogacy arrangements were 'not a good idea' because it was 'like messing with a human body'. His concern focused on the transience of a baby born of a surrogacy agreement and he implicitly compared the procedure with (what he perceived to be) a less complicated 'giving away' of sperm and eggs; better, he argued, 'to keep it simple'.

The preoccupation with the potential difficulties facing surrogate mothers and children born through such arrangements is matched by a concomitant concern for the 'rights' of commissioning parents. The 'heart-ache' suffered by infertile couples and the chance of their having a baby through a surrogate arrangement is not ignored nor forgotten, it is merely displaced when certain questions are being addressed. When surrogacy is addressed from the perspective of commissioning parties who also provide the genetic material, then their claim as parents through the genetic link is acknowledged. Alan pointed out that if he and his wife had needed fertility treatment and had 'donated – it would still be our child even though it has been carried by someone else'. He had told me on a previous occasion he would not consider donating sperm. He argued vehemently that any children born from his sperm would be his and that link could never be severed:

> You'd feel connected – you are! The thought of having a child some-where and not knowing, and [not] knowing it's Okay.

Relatives appropriated through marriage (step or 'half' relatives as well as affines) or relatives created through adoption, while no less real in their existence are thought not to be 'real' in their identity as relatives; are not, in other words, fully related.[7] It is recognised that 'half' relatives (those connected by substance through one avenue rather than two) have a more tenuous claim on relatedness than do 'full' relatives. A young woman told me she was 'very close' to her stepbrother (her mother's son from a second marriage). She argued that she would be extremely upset at any suggestion that he were any less than fully related.

> I can talk to him; there's a bond there even though he is my *step-*brother – mind you, I wouldn't let anybody say that and get away with it.

During fieldwork, I was invited to participate in an adult creative writing class which comprised an English teacher and between six and eight Alltown women, between 40 and 72 years of age. In one of my discussions with the class, Mrs Allen, referring to her daughter by a first marriage, argued forcefully that her daughter had not been brought up 'step-anything'.[8] She believes many of the problems inherent in step-families were attenuated in her family because her daughter disliked her 'real' father and 'the whole of his family'; consequently, she experienced no conflict of loyalty between them and her stepfather. She went on to reflect that from a mother's point of view, it did not matter where the 'seed' came from, it was always your child. This leads her to question whether, in fact, being a stepchild *has* had an effect on her daughter:

> [S]he's always had a chip on her shoulder. She's 50 now so she should have more sense. She's still got a big chip on her shoulder feeling that she's been an outcast, but she hasn't – never. She's always been treated just like the others.

These thoughts prompted another member of the group, Mrs Eaves, to add that she has always felt slightly jealous of the unity she perceives between her mother, stepfather and step-siblings (the children of her mother and stepfather). As she put it:

> I don't know, I think sometimes you have that feeling though. You know I have a brother and sister who are true stepbrothers and sisters. And you get a little bit jealous of that closeness that they had.

In this quotation, we see a differentiation appearing between degrees of step-siblings. In Mrs Eaves's view, the children of a mother and stepfather are more truly step than the children of, one assumes, a stepfather's previous marriage. Her poignant remarks present a model of two parents, each contributing to the unique child and thus forging links which comprise a 'family unit'. She perceives that being linked through just one side of the equation diminishes her claim to belong. Paula Seddon has two teenage sons by a previous marriage. Stuart Seddon describes his role as stepfather:

> It is difficult to be a stepfather. David is close to Paula. If he was in trouble you'd help and pretend he was your own.

Later, talking about sperm donation, Stuart suggested that most men who had a child conceived through donor insemination would 'pretend there was a connection'. Although, he went on, 'it would always be in the back of your mind that it is not your child.' Mrs Seddon, Stuart's mother (whom I spoke with separately) explained that although her husband was not, in fact, the 'true' grandfather of the younger children (being Stuart's stepfather), he nevertheless considered Stuart's children 'more his grandchildren than his real grandchildren' whom he rarely saw.

An interrelated distinction is made, then, between full and half relatives and between blood relatives and those appropriated through marriage or adoption. This is evident in the emphasis people place on 'accepting' step- or adopted children 'as if' they were 'their own'. And while the onus is on the older generation to accept children who enter families in this way, it is also the case that children are seen to have a will and an intention in setting the tone of the relationship.

LINKS THAT MEDIATE

PC: [T]he other thing is, Jan, it's like love binds families together and I do consciously take time out to go around and tell everybody about what everybody else is doing because the others don't visit one another. I'm the only person that sees *all* my brothers and sisters. Some of my . . .

JE: So you're like the gatekeeper?

PC: Yeah, I'm like the connector, yeah. I'm like the intercessor for them. My brother —— and my brother —— they've got bloody bicker- ments and arguments now, that they bloody had in the playground. And they are, like, nearly 40 year old.

When I asked Patrick Croft (PC) about the donation of eggs and sperm and the implications of donors being either anonymous or related to the recipi- ent, he pointed out that we were now into 'the realms' of his family, as that, in a way, was 'exactly' what had happened with him. Patrick modelled the problems he perceives to be inherent in NRT on his own experiences of kinship: he was brought up to believe his mother was his sister and his grandmother his mother. He considers both the children of his mother and her husband (Patrick's stepfather) and the children (both younger and older than himself) of his grandmother to be his siblings. None of his siblings, he says, are *full* brothers and sisters. In talking about possibilities presented in assisted reproduction, he talks about relationships. His con- cern was that children conceived through such techniques could be presented with similar kinds of problems he faced in categorising his kin. Patrick also remarked on how relieved he is to know that he was not conceived through an 'incestuous relationship'.

Key kinsfolk may connect a person to their past, or they may mediate between kin who would otherwise not communicate. Paula Seddon describes her sadness at the death of her mother's sister in terms of the loss of somebody who knew, and could tell her, about past family ties: 'She was a touch with the past.' Links to past relatives are also rendered visible in a common notion that genetic traits 'skip a generation', so that characteristics from grandparents are as likely, if not more likely, to be manifest in children as those from parents. Grandmothers (I speak of grandmothers because it is from grandmothers rather than grandfathers that I collected these views) consider themselves to be directly related to their grandchildren. They described grandchildren as 'their own'; they 'belong' to them. The link is mediated by a son or daughter and while a grandchild is a unique person made up from the combination of two sets of inheritance, the affinal set is suspended for this purpose. Affines are perceived to be 'not really' family while grandchildren are indisputably so.

Mrs Seddon (Paula's husband's mother) reflects on her relationship with her grandchildren. She thinks she has not had the opportunity to be a grandmother to Paula's two older sons but considers the two 'little ones' as 'her own'. (She realises that this view of 'ownership' is a potential source of conflict between her and her son. As we shall see, similar conflicts are raised as possibilities when people discuss mother to daughter or sister to sister egg donation – fears are expressed that such practices may lead to mothers or sisters having additional claims on grandchildren or nieces and nephews, thereby upstaging the parents and threatening the existing relationship between mother and daughter or sister and sister.) She points out that Paula's older sons have a set of relatives on their father's side whom she does not know, leading her to conclude that she can never fully 'know' the boys. While the existence of bilateral kin ties is acknowledged in her views on relatedness, they are not activated when she describes her link to her younger grandchildren, which is unequivocal and mediated by her son.

Mary Greenwood was invited to think about whom she would include as 'family'. She thinks she should include her daughters-in-law; after all, she points out:

> [T]hem lasses have both said, when they were married: 'Do you know, we can always come and talk to you, can always talk to you better than anybody else; we can come and tell you us problems.' So, really I must have accepted them as family mustn't I? If they felt like that; if they felt they could come to me with their problems.

Mary describes an affective relationship between family members but she goes on to make a distinction between that and relatedness. The difference is made visible, she argues, through feelings; her daughters-in-law do not, she says, evoke the same 'flip flop' feeling in her as do her sons and her grandchildren:

> Wives don't belong like [the] lads do. I don't get that glow – it's a different sort of glad feeling when I see them.

Having said that, Mary is aware of, and sensitive to, the needs of maintaining and encouraging the link between herself and her daughters-in-law by playing down qualitative differences in her feelings, but it is clear she perceives her connection to her grandchildren to lie through her sons. And presented with a hypothetical example, supposing that her daughters-in-law had children from previous marriages, Mary hopes and believes she would have tried extremely hard to accept them 'as if they were her own'.

People are concerned to treat those they perceive as not 'fully' related as if they were. Making distinctions between 'step' and 'real' differentiates between two types of relatedness. However, this is counter-productive when the unity of 'family' is at stake. Difference may be denied, but of course it is in denial that differentiation lies.

Disrupting links

Assistance is supposed to flow from older to younger generations. While parents should help children, the same strength of expectation is not held for children toward their parents (Finch 1989; Strathern 1991b). In this context, one might consider the fact that daughter to mother egg donation is thought to be more problematic than mother to daughter. As one woman put it:

> It's like messing with generations, like an erupting volcano; it would drive a wedge between them. It's a special relationship – the mother – daughter bond. That bond would be altered – you'd lose the law of mother and daughter relations . . . plonking a baby in the middle takes all the laws away.

This quotation makes a negative point about the way children mediate links between kinsfolk. Here, mediation acts to stop the flow; it acts as an obstruction in the line between mother and daughter.

Concerns generated by thoughts of mother/daughter egg substitution focus not only on appropriate flows of assistance and on unobstructed links, but also on sexual relations. Veronica Thomas, in her early twenties and married (to Alan), asserted that a daughter could only donate an egg to her mother if certain criteria were met. First, her mother's partner must be her stepfather; second, she should never have lived in the same household as her mother and partner; third, she must have lived away from home for at least six years before the onset of the relationship between her mother and stepfather. This fairly embracing set of rules was presented with seemingly little premeditation; I note that it precludes men who might act in the role of father with or without a genetic link.

Daughters donating eggs to their mothers is regarded, by most people, as perplexing in a special way. It is visualised as a question of the egg from a daughter being introduced to sperm from her father. The unease people feel about mother and daughter egg substitution is thus located not only in ideas about the reversal or 'mixing up' of inter-generational expectations, but also in ideas about crossing boundaries into incestuous relationships between fathers and their daughters. Similarly, brothers donating sperm to sisters or sisters donating eggs to brothers, a possibility raised by one person and pursued by others, evoked incest immediately. The important thing is not that the union of their gametes sets up a relationship between the two, but that their relatedness is a fact prior to the union; that is, there is already a connection between the gametes.

Alltown people represent the conception of children, in the context of NRTs, on an 'as if' there were a sexual relationship model, but only where there are prior kinship ties. Hence people do not make an analogy, in the case of a child conceived through the anonymous donation of gametes, between fertilisation in vitro and fertilisation through sex. Yet immediately the issue of kinship enters the equation, then incest is raised as a limiting factor.

Discussions about sister to sister egg donation generate two seemingly opposing views that echo the general viewpoints people take on the NRT as a whole. One emphasises the advantages and the other highlights the dangers of such a practice.

The first view focuses on the idea that sisters are the 'closest' of kin, which would make the substitution of their gametes unproblematic, or at least less problematic than in other transfers. There are two interrelated premises to this argument: first, that sisters have closely resembling ova; and second, that sisters will be more willing to assist each other than unrelated women. The perceived similarity in gamete material, the argument goes, enables genes to be kept 'within the family' so that the ensuing offspring will be constituted of as near the genetic make-up of its parents as possible. The advantage of substituting eggs from a sister rather than from an anonymous donor is thus conceptualised through perceived similarities between sisters and the concept of shared substance. One woman took this to its logical conclusion and supposed the ideal egg donor to be a Siamese twin.

The second view focuses on the threat that sister to sister egg donation poses to existing relationships. Two main disruptions are predicted, one between the sisters themselves and the other between the donating sister and her brother-in-law (the father of the child). It is argued that the donating sister will feel a greater attachment or claim to the child than is usual or appropriate for a mother's sister. It is thought she will have a 'special relationship' with the child which could either be a positive or destructive influence; it could add to the child's life – two mothers are better than one, or else the child could lose out and instead of gaining a mother, lose an aunt. People predict that the donor may be more tempted to 'interfere' in the child's upbringing, thus usurping the privileges of parents and causing conflict. Even grandparents who think of their grandchildren as 'their own' note a difference in their relationship with grandchildren as opposed to their children: an often-heard comment is that they can always 'give them back'. Thus while caring and wanting the best for their grandchildren, grandparents recognise that ultimate responsibility lies with parents. Interference in child-rearing has the potential for causing conflict between sisters and endangering their relationship.

While kin relationships are on the one hand thought to be enduring – you can always choose your friends but not your family – they are on the other hand also thought to be fragile, easily disrupted and require great patience and tenacity to sustain in an appropriate manner.

Creating links that were not there

An important consideration raised in the transfer of eggs between sisters was, as I have noted, the relationship between the donating sister and the father of the child (her brother-in-law). This relationship is created through marriage and hence can be dissolved on divorce; an in-law can become an ex-in-law, whereas a sister does not usually become an ex-sister even if all communication and contact is broken – sisters remain sisters. The introduction to the sister and brother-in-law relationship of a child has the potential for creating a different kind of relationship, one mediated by conception.

It is often remarked that ideally children should be born within a 'loving relationship'. That loving relationship is also thought to be forged through the conception of a child; a bond between parents may grow stronger, or be created, in sharing responsibility for the creation and care of another human being. So while, as one young Alltown man said, 'two parts joined together make a child' (he might have added a unique child), it is not merely gametes that make children. Making children also requires a relationship between the parents. There are similar implications when eggs and sperm are fertilised in vitro; a bond could be forged between, in this case, a woman's sister (the egg donor) and her husband. In effect, an adulterous liaison is envisaged. But it is not merely adulterous (implying the setting up of a relationship as if it were sexual, thereby betraying a spouse); it goes further in so far as it embraces the relationship between parents and children. While it is obvious that parents create children, it is less obvious, but no less true, that children create parents. The birth of a child has the potential for creating parents not only out of its parents but out of the donating woman and, in the case of sister egg donation, her sister's husband. This is thought to pose a threat, not only to the existing tie between spouses, but also to that between sisters.[9]

The topic of sperm donation focuses on similar problems but with a different emphasis: here, it is the competitiveness between males in reproduction which features large in both men's and women's ideas about sperm substitution. It is thought that men would be less willing to receive sperm donated from their brothers, and more willing to make use of sperm donated anonymously. Generally, men are thought to be able to cope less well with the knowledge that their brother is 'the father' of their child. The contrast is that, between sisters, gamete donation has the potential for creating a closer tie, whereas between brothers it is more likely to cause conflict. If eggs are transferred between sisters, and fertilisation modelled on sexual intercourse, then 'the union' is conceptualised as if it were between a woman's husband and her sister. In brother to brother sperm donation, the union would be between a man's wife and his brother. The latter is generally thought to be the more problematic.[10] This might be analysed in terms of underlying gender distinctions in so far as there are gender differences in the implications of sexual infidelity (note how many more cuckolds there are than cuckqueans[11]). Men are assumed to be more proprietorial in their sexual relationships and less tolerant than women of the infidelity of partners. While this is clearly not the case, discussion of gender stereotypes is beyond the scope of this chapter.

Children grow up, and adults look back: in retrospect, stepchildren may consider themselves to have always been on the fringes of the 'real' family. A further example of retrospective reasoning was given by a young man who described to me the importance of 'roots' to children. All children, he noted, liked to look at photographs; in so doing they place their relatives and 'see' how they are related. Children, however, who are conceived through donor insemination or through surrogacy arrangements would be unable to trace their 'roots' in this way; connections made visible in photographs would be absent. To look to the past in order to explain a current concern is a commonly evoked form of evidence, of which there are numerous examples in this chapter. Indeed, the notion that knowledge rests in the recesses of one's mind comes up again and again in discussions about NRTs. Parents of children born from donated gametes, it is argued, will always know the facts of the child's conception and how such knowledge will emerge at a later date or the effect that it will have on relationships is unpredictable.

Time is an important factor in this conceptualisation, so that what may be understood, accepted and agreed upon at one moment in time may be doubted and be the cause of conflict in the future. As one man pointed out:

'It's all right saying, Right, I'll do this thing now with love and honesty and with truth, but you get in an argument with somebody and that goes out of the window.'

The truth, then, will emerge when one least expects it; genetic traits will eventually surface, and 'niggling doubts' will manifest themselves. Secrets have a nasty habit of being disclosed when least expected and, so it is said, the truth will always out.

ROOTS: FIXING AND DIFFERENTIATING

Names locate a person in a nexus of kin. The following excerpt taken from a discussion with members of the creative writing class illustrates the problems people are faced with when there is ambiguity in kin terms.

SM: And I don't know. I don't know whether it's soon enough to know – I don't know what differences these odd situations make in families and neighbourhoods. I remember having a discussion here some time ago, when this unemployed workers' centre was started – actually it was at the baths – the question was what do you call the man, y'know. People had always talked about their husbands or 'him at home' or whatever . . .

M: Well now they call them their live-in lover don't they or their boyfriend?

SM: And you've got to have a new term . . .

M: Or their toy boy . . . I could do with one of them.
      Laughter

SM: So it's the same.

J: We should be so lucky Molly!

SM: And there was this laddie in the Watch Group. I knew his mother and his father . . . no I knew his mother's boyfriend, I think he was – I don't think she'd remarried – and himself, and I would always forget that this wasn't his father – he would come and act like his father, y'know. And I would say: Has your father got one of these? Then I'd think, Oh now – has . . . and I'd have to think, has . . . and I'd have to use his Christian name, you know? I knew his Christian name anyway and would use it, but normally when you talk to children you don't use the father's Christian name – you say your father. I had to slip into this and er . . . there's a lot of families that are like that now. So you know there is bound to be some sort of difference in the aura of things, in a way.

Like Mrs Seddon who speculates that, had her step-grandchildren called her and her husband 'grandma' and 'grandpa', there would have been a difference in the quality of their relationship, so Mrs Moore (SM) perceives there to be an inevitable difference in 'the aura' of things when kin terms are not used in expected ways.

Unattached gametes present people with similar conceptual problems. In a discussion with two women, Lucy Davis and Theresa Lee, both in their early thirties, and neighbours, friends and work partners, I raised the issue of gamete donation and the preservation of embryos by freezing. Theresa had previously noted that she would, had the need arisen, have considered donating an egg to Lucy. However, both women found the idea of using gametes from anonymous donors problematic. Lucy, after much thought, said she could not 'see anonymous donations'. She went on to argue that 'they should have a name and address on every egg and sperm', so if they *needed* to freeze eggs, at least 'they would be safe in her [the donor's] name'. Her comments centre on the danger of unattached gametes; while possessing the donor's name, she argues, they still 'belong' to her. Here, the idiom of ownership implies a relationship.'[12] By contrast, when Lucy and Theresa express a reluctance to allow scientists or clinicians ownership of gamete material, ownership in this context denies a relationship. They go on to predict the potential for misuse; a use that benefits only 'the scientist' without reference to social responsibility. However, if gametes remain connected by name to the donor, before being re-embodied and identified with the recipient, then social responsibility is seen to prevail.

Naming acts, on the one hand, to differentiate – it gives voice to variability – while on the other hand, it aggregates – making the connections between people conspicuous. Naming the baby itself was raised as a problem in discussions about surrogacy: should it have the surrogate mother's [sur]name, asked one man, or 'the sperm's'? For names are thought to do more than merely label people in a convenient shorthand; they are said to affect the aura of things and alter the quality of relationships. Above all, they attach persons to specific others and in the case of the vulnerable gamete or baby would fix them to persons in a way that is thought to render them safe from manipulation.

It is those attachments that also give persons their unique characteristics. Variability between persons is thought to stem not only from a particular constellation of kin but also from gestation and birth experiences, and from primary feeding relationships. For example, Veronica Thomas described how confident both her children are. She explains this with reference to early feeding relationships: her husband, she says, played a role in looking after their son when he was born, feeding him and taking him out in the pushchair, whereas he 'ignored' their daughter until she was about

12 months old. However, Veronica breast-fed her daughter and as a consequence she feels the child is now equally as confident as her brother.

I noted at the beginning of this chapter that the Alltown people whose views about NRT I elicited were, for the most part, intrigued by the topic and were interested in it beyond our immediate interactions. Hence, Mary Greenwood was reminded of my research in a letter to Marjorie Proops she read in a magazine (see above); Paula Seddon called me to tell me of a breakfast-time television discussion about the possibility of post-menopausal women achieving pregnancy through technological assistance, and another woman cut out and presented me with a letter to Dr Miriam Stoppard published in a magazine and entitled, 'Can first cousins get married?'[13] My initial conversations with Alltown residents prompted some people to think further about other implications and possibilities of reproductive medicine, which they raised in conversation, unelicited, at a later date.

Several days after discussing with me the advantages and potential problems in donor insemination, Veronica raised the possibility that children could be 'brought into the world by scientists . . . without any real beginnings or real ancestors or family'. She went on to predict the effects of babies reared in a laboratory:

> Somebody somewhere must be creating this artificial womb. A baby reacts to what you're feeling – if your heartbeat is faster then the baby's heartbeat is faster. It could be fed on just vegetables – how would it react then, through the placenta – not what you fancy like crisps, or salad, or Chewitts on the bus, like cravings at different times – vegetables, sweets, alcohol whatever it takes to make a baby. It will have no feelings because no feelings are going through it.

It is variation that makes persons. In these remarks, Veronica is concerned with the developing tie between a mother and child. The placenta mediates the relationship and the placenta comprises shared substance. Variation and spontaneity in the mother's diet is thought to have an effect, through the placenta, on the child's development, as do emotions such as hatred, anger and love which emanate from the mother and pass also through the placenta. Exposure to such emotions has an effect on the fetus: without that exposure, the fetus itself will not develop feelings or emotions. A controlled diet at controlled times – a lack of variability and spontaneity running through the placenta – will produce uniform people; people without feelings. Veronica is arguing that a lack of different stimuli will diminish variability between persons. This danger may also be represented in the idiom of 'cloning'. The following two examples show how the notion of 'cloning' came up in conversation and how it portrays, again, a boundary to the technological intervention in human reproduction.

Keith Davis expressed his concern about the way a child born through a surrogacy arrangement should be named thus:

> Whose name in a surrogate motherhood goes on the birth certificate? Is it the father? . . . must be the father of the sperm [if] only because of the laws of the land. But who's the mother? If the egg has come . . . if the egg has been donated, then surely the woman who gives birth must be classed as the mother.

He went on to predict that in 'fifteen years' time' such a concern might be irrelevant because 'from DNA they will be able to create matter'. He argued that DNA is, in a sense, 'another form of sperm and eggs', and added that in the media 'we've already been talking about cloning'.

One Alltown woman expressed concerns about NRT in terms of the way that intervention entailed a pre-arranged or pre-organised element. She explained: 'I would hate to grow up thinking that that was what my background was; that I'd been organised through different bodies and pre-arranged.' She continued:

> I started off by saying where I started off in life and I mentioned class, didn't I? Now today I don't think of class. I think now that, you know, I'm as good as anybody else and anybody else is as good as me. And I like to think that everybody's got a fairly reasonable chance in life to make what they will of it for themselves. But if it was all sort of prearranged, they'd *clone* us so that we had – we'd have a group of workers, and a group, you know, of people giving orders and so on and so on and you'd never get the chance to move out of that. . . . You wouldn't have the chance to – in my view you wouldn't then have the chance to make worthwhile relationships and affections. We'd just all be *zombies*. [Emphasis added.]

Ideas about 'cloning' are put forward when people attempt to place a limit on the scientific endeavour. Again, the notion need not be interpreted as an overly-anxious response to technological progress but rather as an expression of knowledge about what constitutes a person.

No two people share an exact replica of the two pasts which constitute an individual and if they do (as in the case of siblings), then time of birth, position in sibling order, or early feeding experiences can all be given as examples of experiences which differentiate between unique individuals. It is assumed that much forethought and planning is required for people to go through forms of assisted conception or surrogacy arrangements. While it is the control of unpredictability and spontaneity in human reproduction that is, in this context, questionable, the 'medical danger' of other practices, such as anonymous gamete donations, focuses instead on the unpredictable. Several people, on different occasions, argued that not knowing the genetic 'make-up' of a child will present problems when compiling adequate and appropriate medical records. It is considered important for the future well-being of children that medical histories of parents and grandparents (rarely, I think, do we consult more distant ancestors) are included in their own. On the one hand, then, removing randomness in reproduction is thought to be undesirable; on the other hand, there is a concern that unpredictable characteristics may manifest themselves in the child. What indeed, pointed out one woman, will happen if a donor is a 'bad 'un'? It is thought that parents are less likely to tolerate problematic characteristics if the child is not 'their own', if, in other words, they do not think of themselves as ultimately responsible either for the particular characteristic or indeed for the child.

Analogies with adoption are made with a different emphasis again. Here, the child for 'its own good' must be told the facts; if not, there is a strong likelihood that the 'facts' will emerge at a later date. Many stories are told and examples given of people finding out, usually as adults, that they had been adopted as children. It is considered impossible to keep such information secret; neighbours, relatives, friends may tell inadvertently or maliciously. At the same time, people talk of the inevitability of children wishing to 'trace their roots'; there are stories of how adopted people go to great lengths to trace their 'real' parents and such stories often touch on the anguish this may cause adoptive parents.

Consider the following, again from the creative writing class:

SM: Well, I mean, we're talking about scientific things now but my uncle was adopted, for instance, and I don't know how much he wondered about his real mother but his adopted mother was always his mother from his point of view. As far as the family was concerned um . . . it's more to do with relationships than it is to do with birth, I think; and the relationships what you build up. And I had a discussion with me mother some time ago and something to the effect that it wasn't blood necessarily that counted, it was the relationship that you'd built up between you, which I think does count for more. But that can always be disturbed by, as you say, adopted people growing up and wondering and trying to find out where they actually came from: which I can imagine will also take place with those who want to find out what laboratory . . .

MB: They want to know their origins, don't they?

SM: Because they feel somehow they belong somewhere and . . .

MB: And they want to know which box they slot into. It's funny that, isn't it?

This excerpt takes us back to a fundamental conceptualisation that persons are located in time and place through their kin connections, as well as to the tension between social and biological parenting. As Mrs Brierley (MB) puts it, people 'want to know which box they slot into'; their unique nexus of relations differentiates theirs from everybody else's.

Roots fix a person on branches linking kinsfolk; it is not necessary to have known them, but one should know of them. A link with the past is conceptualised through past relatives and knowing of them locates a person in time and place. This location is fixed, and at first glance appears to counterpoise the infinite variability of persons which elsewhere is so positively valued. In fact, of course, such seemingly fixed positions in networks of kin *constitute* infinite variability. Each person is rooted in a unique location relative to their kinsfolk: they are not free-floating individuals.

CONCLUSION: WHAT KIND OF CONCERNS?

Veronica was one of the first people in Alltown with whom I discussed NRT. I have noted how she commented on the implications and predicted the outcome of combining gametes, in vitro and in utero, from a variety of sources. She talked of the advantages and disadvantages of using gametes first of all from anonymous and then from known donors, and she predicted the problems that could arise in each of these practices. Her immediate ability to present numerous possibilities and to embed the possibilities within a variety of scenarios, without apparent forethought, influenced the questions I went on to ask of other people in the town.

Alltown people whose views are presented here recognise a plurality of perspectives and have no difficulty in attributing to others differing opinions on similar topics; the differences are thought to depend on all kinds of social criteria, which they summarise as 'depending on the person'. This returns me to a point made at the beginning of this chapter: it is sometimes assumed that the role of the anthropologist is to uncover popular understanding or 'public opinion'. But, as we have seen, there is no one view on reproductive technology any more than there is a single public opinion. Instead there is a veritable variety of perspectives. In this chapter, the perspectives do not comprise simple positions that correspond to people's social standing or experience. Instead I have pointed to the way the standpoint taken depends on the question being addressed and the reason for addressing it.

Certain dangers preoccupy people when they explore the implications of assisted conception. These dangers, although interlinked, may be placed into three main categories which I shall call psychological, biological and relational.

Psychological dangers arise when people talk about potential future effects of, for example, donor insemination or surrogacy arrangements on children born through such procedures. The danger is perceived to be particularly acute if all attempt has been made to hide the facts of birth from the child and the story emerges later in life. Idioms such as 'screwed up' or 'drop outs' are used to describe the effects of discovery, or the feeling of difference that such children may experience. This danger I have related to common notions that the 'truth' will emerge and that knowledge, like matter, cannot be destroyed. Biological dangers are related to what are perceived to be genetic risks when particular categories of kin reproduce; restricting the pool of genes is thought to result in complex genetic problems. Idioms of 'interbreeding' are commonly evoked as evidence of the biological dangers inherent in NRT. These can be related to ideas about distance and closeness, including those which arise in the English penchant for constructing difference through suggestions that 'other' places (however near) are hotbeds of 'interbreeding'.

The dangers which I call psychological and biological are familiar and feature in public discussion about NRT. The third is raised constantly by Alltown people but appears to be less salient in parliamentary debates or clinical assessments. It concerns the way in which potential and possible practices in NRT will affect social relationships. The dangers posed to existing relationships are rendered visible in ideas put forward about ambivalent kinship roles, conflicting claims on children and 'interference' in relationships which ought to be enduring. Technological intervention could disrupt existing relationships or create novel, but antagonistic, relationships.

These three dangers are linked in a commonly expressed disquiet about the 'power' of the medical and scientific professions. In this context, people make analogies between, for example, scientists and God, or scientists and Hitler. These analogies suggest that science has overstepped the mark, and that limits need to be placed on technological innovation. From the perspective of a different interest group, such remarks may be interpreted as uninformed or even Luddite reactions to technological change. Such an interpretation assumes that given further information (of the right kind) people will understand the technologies better and, in so doing, will be less anxious about their implications. This argument treats anxieties and ideas about boundaries as if they referred only to techniques of reproductive assistance and were somehow isolated from the wider context in which they are generated. If, however, we attempt to understand how the dangers listed above are interrelated and if, at the same time, we look at the contexts in which they arise, then it is possible to understand fears not as idiosyncratic views but informed by, and part of, a system of ideas.

The several people in Alltown whom I invited to talk about NRT were intrigued by the topic; they were not only interested in the issues but keen to talk about them, a point we had not predicted prior to the fieldwork. Indeed, one brief we set ourselves was to discover what questions might elicit information about relatedness and in which contexts. The Alltown people quoted in this chapter were prepared to respond to many issues raised simply as topics or hypothetical scenarios. In that sense, they presented us with ways of questioning, as well as with their answers. They discussed the implications of assisted conception with authority and insight, as well as with empathy towards those who require fertility services.

People interpret what they see as the implications of NRT not through what they know of the techniques and philosophies of reproductive medicine, but through what they know about the practice and predictabilities of kinship. They do not, in other words, have to be technologically literate in the methods of NRT in order to think about the implications of certain reproductive possibilities for the social relationships they create and/or influence. The Alltown people whose views are presented here ground their ideas about NRT in what they already know and, indeed, in what they are expert at.

NOTES

1 A commonly used Alltown idiom.
2 La Fontaine (1988: 15) concludes: 'Incest is not merely a symbolic violation of kinship but the sexual abuse of children.' It should be noted that my references to incest are of a different order than the excruciatingly difficult concern with cases of child abuse that informs La Fontaine's discussion. I am not looking at cases of incest. My interest has been on how people talk about kinship in the light of NRT, and incest frequently comes up when certain possibilities are explored.
3 Because the speaker had three young children to contend with while pregnant.
4 In a completely different context, prior to this study, one Alltown woman talking about 'family' said: 'Maybe [we] shouldn't expect so much from them – they're just people. Some friends are more family than family.'
5 While many of the Alltown people with whom I spoke recognised that women might be motivated to act as surrogates for altruistic reasons, a disquiet was often expressed as to what the 'real' reasons might be. One

woman listed the 'types' of women she foresaw as wanting to act as host surrogates: first, there are those who want 'to be helpful'; second, those who may be 'a bit insecure' and crave 'the attention' one gets when pregnant; third, 'lady scientists' who for experimental purposes will want to know 'whether it can be done'.

6 Lucy Davis (LD) insisted I (JE) interview her husband (KD) as she thought it would not only be interesting but also as a 'technical person' (he is an engineer) and a man, he would think and talk differently about NRT than she and her friend had done. A meeting was arranged which, falling on Keith's birthday, was relocated to a pub and Lucy was persuaded to join us. The following excerpt took place two hours into the conversation after certain possibilities of IVF by donor and surrogacy had been discussed (see text). It indicates not only Lucy's interest in the subject but also the way Keith perceives my role as 'drawing out' the relevant information; in other words, in asking the right questions.

LD: It's so interesting. I've told everyone I know about it . . .
KD: One thing I've just thought of . . . How do the children feel?
LD: Well, me, Theresa and Jeanette have gone into all this, we've gone much further into depth about this, look[ed] at it socially.
KD: Well, why haven't I?
JE: We were getting there.
LD: We were five hours, me, Theresa and Jeanette; we had more chance to delve into it deeper.
KD: Well, why haven't I, then?
JE: I think that is a good question though [about the children].
KD: Especially in the surrogacy part of it . . .

7 My interest is not in eliciting differences in the relationships between step and 'real' parents and relating this to, for example, family arrangements (La Fontaine 1985), but rather in how differences are conceptualised within a wider model of relatedness.

8 In their discussion of kinship in a 'middle-class sector of London', Firth *et al.* write: 'in the English kinship system terms of address are not merely stereotyped linguistic labels, but are dynamic expressions of attitudes and relationships' (1969: 338).

9 We are reminded of a parliamentary debate at the turn of the century which turned on similar perceptions of threat, namely the debate about whether a man should be allowed to marry his dead wife's sister (Wolfram 1987). Referring to Wolfram's discussion of the controversy, La Fontaine (1990) points out that similar arguments were later used in discussions about the function of the incest taboo. During fieldwork, a report in a local newspaper described the marriage of a man to his deceased wife's mother. Several Alltown residents with whom I spoke were reminded of this when considering the implications of sperm and egg donations. Although it was argued by one woman that it was 'not incestuous' as a man is 'not related to his mother-in-law', she was nevertheless perplexed about such a union. The newspaper had portrayed the marriage as an altruistic act of benefit to the child of the man and his deceased wife and had emphasised the fact that the child would be 'brought up' by someone who knew and loved her (her

grandmother). The familiar argument of 'keeping it in the family' was used. Yet the women who mentioned this report to me were sceptical of this representation and questioned the motives of the newly married couple. Their anxiety appeared to focus partly on the conflation of the identity of grandmother and stepmother and partly on what they saw as the 'betrayal' of the deceased woman, but in the context of reproductive technology it would seem to be the concept of 'keeping it in the family' which causes concern.

10 Haimes (1991) discusses the ways in which sperm and egg donations and donors were perceived and judged differently by members of the Warnock Committee (cf. Chapter 1).

11 See Mills (1991) for an interesting note about the disappearance of cuckquean from common English usage.

12 When I call my brother 'our Billy', I am not implying that I, or indeed we, own him: by labelling him in such possessive terms, I identify him, *through his relationship to me*, from all the other Billys there might be.

13 Towards the end of my fieldwork in Alltown, the controversy about single women being offered IVF (so-called 'virgin births') erupted in the newspapers. Although the comments I heard about this issue again reflected the general debate on reproductive technology, in so far as the positive and negative aspects of such a practice were raised, the 'controversy' exercised people much less than might have been predicted. There seemed to me, at the time, to be a decided lack of interest or concern in the issue compared to the interest people had shown in the impact of surrogacy and gamete donation on kinship. And while the familiar argument arose that children born through IVF by donor would have difficulty tracing their roots, the following comment seems to encapsulate the relative lack of concern about single women having access to assisted conception: 'I can't imagine many women wanting to have a child before, you know, doing it.' 'Virgin births' appear to be seen more as an individual and idiosyncratic choice and less relevant to wider issues of kinship than other forms of reproductive intervention. While this point merits further exploration, I raise it in this chapter to indicate that Alltown people are not intrigued by all aspects of NRT in the same way.

Afterword for Chapter 2
Clones – who are they?

Jeanette Edwards

A point still made in social scientific commentary on new reproductive and genetic technologies is that they present nothing new. This argument has it that people (cultures) are infinitely adaptable and the 'biological facts' of human reproduction are already assimilated and 'represented' in all kinds of different ways across the world. From such a vantage point, technological intervention in conception presents just another innovation in the many and diverse ways in which human societies create and constitute persons and social relationships. Kinship, from this perspective, is an infinitely malleable and 'plastic' institution.

Revisiting this chapter, I see why it might have been used to exemplify how 'ordinary people' assimilate the new and the technological to what they already, 'traditionally', know. After all, I stated (perhaps too baldly) that the people with whom I worked in Alltown 'model new possibilities on old facts', and they 'ground their ideas about NRT in what they already know', but this should not imply that nothing has changed. Concepts such as assimilation or adaptation are inadequate to explain the ways in which people, with no vested interest in NRT, explore them with reference to what they know about the reproduction of persons and social relationships. And conversely, the way in which they explore what it means to be related in a focus on NRT. If assisted conception is apprehended through the cultural lens of kinship, then kinship is apprehended through that of assisted conception. In this mutually constitutive process, neither ideas about kinship nor NRT are fixed or immutable.

The chapter on which this afterword reflects shows how Alltown people draw on their own experiences of intimate relationships to reflect on consequences of novel practices of which they have no experience. It also demonstrates the ways in which people hypothesise from what we might call cultural theories about the reproduction of persons, and how they reflect upon what they know about how individuals, families and other collectivities are constituted. Veronica Thomas, for example, theorises that a human being created in a laboratory (perhaps in an artificial womb) will have a deficit of emotions because they will not have been privy to emotions, via the placenta, during gestation. And Margaret Seddon is sceptical about the benefits that might accrue from 'cloning', predicting that any such techniques will only be used to the advantage of the elite and the disadvantage of many. From certain scientific perspectives, such concerns are dismissed as 'Brave New World' scenarios and born of ignorance. Labelled sometimes as 'public opinion', such views are criticised for neither capturing the complexity of scientific research nor the motivation of scientists. Similarly, the concerns of 'scientists', from certain Alltown perspectives, are dismissed as blinkered and narrow. The view from 'science' is criticised for failing to recognise the complexity of bringing up children and the variety of ways in which late-twentieth-century residents of Britain constitute their families, friends and communities. 'Scientists', from this view, are 'out of touch' with the realities of day-to-day living in a place like Alltown.

It is a nonsense to place such perspectives in opposition to each other and to suggest that they relate, in the former case, to those supportive of science and progress and, in the latter, to those who support, say, 'traditional family values'. This is far too reductionist a premise with which to begin to analyse the numerous ways in which people, both those designated as 'ordinary' as well as those designated as 'scientists', are reminded of the intricacies of social relationships in their exploration of NRT.

I take the opportunity of reiterating three points here. First, the people with whom I spoke made connections not only with what they know about intimate social relationships (kinship), but also with what they know about, for example, membership of a social class, or a place (like Alltown), or living on a housing estate, in a 'semi-detached' or a 'back-to-back', and in the north, rather than the south, of England. When Alltown residents talk of possibilities presented by NRT, they predict their implications for social relationships of all kinds, not only 'family' kinds. Relations between different neighbourhoods, as well as between different 'types' of resident, emerge in commentaries about the implications of assisted conception. Alltown people remarked on the stigma attached to both infertility, as well as the stigma attached to the means of overcoming it. They point out that both childlessness and making use of fertility services attract attention. And attention comes not only from friends, neighbours and relatives, but also from associates and other townsfolk, known and unknown.

Second, the so-called 'facts' people mobilise in their commentary on NRT are not items of information which can be retrieved and deployed in order to exemplify a particular point, and then returned intact. Knowledge is itself construed in the process of discursive exploration. Analogies, for example, between NRT and adoption, incest, and 'step' families, do more than incorporate NRT into pre-existing sets of ideas. They also augment as well as diminish those ideas. Understandings of adoption, for example, are expanded by adding comparisons between it and, say, surrogate mother-hood, but they are also diminished as other comparisons are *not* made. Adoption becomes a different kind of option when the possibility (per-ceived or practiced) is available of bypassing infertility and having a child connected in a different way through donated gametes or the services of a surrogate mother (see Bartholet 1993). The making of certain connections (between adoption and gamete donation) entails the 'not-making' of others (between adoption and 'step families'). To read the process by which people make sense of assisted conception as assimilation or adaptation, or as merely 'the views' or 'opinions' of a particular population in a specific local-ity in the north of England, is to ignore the silences and to screen out the contradictions, and thus to simplify what is otherwise an interweaving of perspectives.

Third, the model of kinship mobilised by Alltown residents, in 1990, was not *based* on biological connection. This is not to say that biological ties between persons (expressed in idioms of shared blood or genetic inherit-ance and deemed to be 'natural') are insignificant in Alltown understandings of kinship, but to say that ways in which relationships are forged through care and effort, and sustained through will, are equally significant.[1] While the material from Alltown demonstrates that biological connections are indeed integral to kinship thinking, they are not the foundation from which diversity is built. They are but one element in a system which contains at least two component parts. For biology to work as an idiom of relatedness it requires a counterpart, in this case, 'the social'. Similarly 'the social' attains its meaning through its contrast with all that is 'biological'. They may be thought of as two quite different spheres of reality but they are autonomous only conditionally. They rely on each other for their purchase. If the type of 'Western' kinship exemplified in Alltown relies on the *interplay* between 'the social' and 'the biological',[2] then to privilege one, over and above the other, is conducive to a position that is partisan.

Sitting again with Mary Greenwood (MG) at Paula Seddon's (PS) kit-chen table almost eight years after our first conversations about NRT, it is 'cloning' that dominates our conversation. We reflect on changes that have taken place over the intervening years and Mary identifies what she sees as an ever-increasing explicitness surrounding processes and elements of birth.

MG: I mean, years back birth were a miracle, you know? You just knew [that] these things got together. But now all the mystery's gone and its . . .

PS: It will surely all become much more acceptable, won't it? Like, I can remember people talking about test-tube babies and seeing them as being Frankensteins, and now its quite acceptable to have a test-tube baby.

MG: That's right, yes.

JE: Do you think it is? You think it's changed much?

PS: Yeah [*pause*] I think there's more understanding about – you know, the fact that it's not – I think there was always this image – you know, sort of [*inaudible*] in cartoons, in newspapers – of babies in test-tubes, and I think we have a much more proper understanding [now] that it's not like that ...

MG: They put it together, and then transplant it?

PS: That's right, yeah – its *conception* in a test-tube, or whatever. I'm not quite sure [*laughs*].

MG: That's right, they planted it theirselves.

PS: That's right, and the baby grows inside quite naturally. And maybe cloning [*pause*] you only have to say something enough times for people to accept it.

MG: That's right, yeah, because at first they'll only put the good side to it, won't they? And a lot of people will accept it as such ...

PS: I don't think its even that Mary, I just think it's just, if things get mentioned enough times – you know? like swear words ...

MG: It becomes everyday.[3]

Perhaps this is a reminder of the speed at which new concerns eclipse former ones. But, of course, mysteries remain, albeit differently couched, and our conversation turns constantly on questions that 'cloning' raises: 'Clones – who are they?'; 'Will a clone have a birth certificate with the mother and father on?'; 'What is your spirit when you're a clone?'; 'Where would you be on a family tree?'; 'If you eat Dolly would it be like eating mutton rather than lamb?'. This time Paula's two younger children, Neil, now 13 and Harriet, 11 years old, join in. Instead of popping in and out with requests of their own, they hover, drifting between the kitchen table and the television in the front room, dwelling with us for a while when the conversation catches their interest (which, fortunately, appears to be quite often). The topic of 'cloning' intrigues them. They move with alacrity between sheep and people, and Harriet thinks 'it's stingy':

JE: Why is it stingy? You said it was stingy and snide and it wasn't fair.

HS: [*laughs*] Poor little blighter won't have a parent, will it?

PS: You think that's important?

HS: Yeah [*incredulously*].

NS: But y' *have* still got parents.

PS: Have you still got a parent if you're a clone?

NS: Yes. You've got a mother, because they take your egg and then take the whatsit out the person you're cloning and put it into that egg . . .

MG: Do they [use] a female egg for cloning?

JE: They need an egg, yeah.

PS: It's right then, you don't have a parent.

NS: You *do* have a parent . . . well you've got a biological parent, but not as biological as other parents.

Neil and Harriet imagine what it means to be a parent in the context of 'cloning'. For Neil, it is clear that the female who provides the ova (which host the genetic material being reproduced) is a mother – less biological perhaps than if she were to provide genetic material, but a parent nevertheless. Both he and Harriet know that you cannot be a parent to yourself.

Assisted birth, in the context of NRT, reveals how kinship thinking is constantly re-organising and recontextualising itself, but not randomly. NRT, like adoption, or incest, or 'new family forms', adds complexity but within parameters. And those parameters, in this particular English version of kinship, embrace ideas about 'biological' and 'social' connection. While kinship, in this sense, has always been a hybrid, it is neither infinitely 'plastic' nor infinitely 'malleable'. It has also never been 'traditional'.

NOTES

1 Contemporary critiques of formal anthropological kinship theory have identified the imposition of a genealogical model of kinship onto diverse understandings of the reproduction of persons and social relationships (see, for example, Bouquet 1993; Carsten 1995, 1997; Handler 1995; and for a useful overview see Holy 1996). The idea that kinship is always and everywhere based on the social reckoning of biological connection has been debated, and finally dismissed as ethnocentric.

2 What we call elsewhere the interdigitation between biological and social accounts of relatedness (Edwards and Strathern forthcoming).

3 From the transcript of a conversation taped in early 1998.

3 Negotiated limits

Interviews in south-east England

Eric Hirsch

We have recently been reminded that the notion of modernity passed into popular usage during the mid-nineteenth century. It was Baudelaire who characterised the term in the following way: 'Modernity is the transient, the fleeting, the contingent; it is the one half of art, the other being the eternal and the immutable' (cited in Harvey 1989: 10).[1] Although Baudelaire was addressing the emerging conventions of art during this period, his focus on a tension inherent in aesthetic sensibilities is seen to be replicated in wider social and cultural domains.

One side of the modernist tension, as transience, is exemplified in the ever-changing range of commodities produced and available for mass consumption. The values of individual choice in consumerism are part and parcel of the experiences associated with the fleeting and contingent. The sociology of Simmel, for example, and later commentators, is concerned with examining the individual implications of this aspect of modern life in significant detail (cf. Miller 1987). The other side of this tension, what has been referred to as the 'project' of modernity (Habermas), has intellectual origins which can be traced back to the Enlightenment: the intention behind this project was to reveal the 'universal, eternal, and immutable qualities of humanity through the scientific domination of nature, and the development of rational forms of social organization'. However, the desire to 'dominate nature for rational human ends also entailed the simultaneous domination of human beings' (Harvey 1989: 12–13). There is, thus, a fine line to be discerned between the Enlightenment ideals of equality, liberty and democracy and the twentieth-century developments of totalitarianism (cf. Lefort 1986).

An analogous idiom for rendering this modernist tension is characterised as the relationship between the 'individual' and 'society'; that is, between the individual – as transient and contingent – existing in relationship to society – as enduring and transcendent. This model is a core component of Durkheim's sociology and his sociological project (cf. Lukes 1973: 19–22), but it also figures in the mundane, everyday discourse of social and political life. Much recent debate in anthropology, and social and cultural theory more generally, has asked whether this tension is still an apt characterisation of Euro-American cultures; whether it can be transposed onto cultures outside this context (cf. Strathern 1988); or whether it has been trans-figured into what is now referred to as postmodernism. This is a central theme of Strathern's recent essay on late-twentieth-century English kinship (Strathern 1992a). Her essay forms a key point of reference for the analysis which follows.

This chapter is based on discussions with twelve married couples from central London and a Berkshire town. As it turned out, it was aspects of this 'modern condition' which were explored. The discussions, which focused on themes related to the new reproductive technologies (NRTs), evoked a particular set of tensions intrinsic to this modernism. On the one hand, men and women were prepared to accept (to greater or lesser degrees) that technology could be used to 'improve' on biology/nature. On the other hand, the couples could conceive of these improvements as acceptable so long as the changes to 'nature' were true to its principles. In other words, one could 'give nature a helping hand', as in the case of people having difficulty conceiving children, but this help should go to heterosexual couples: the 'natural' context for conceiving children. A parallel with some of the equivocations encountered in Alltown (see Chapter 2) is evident.

In exploring this tension, three recurrent scenarios have emerged from people's visions. In each of these scenarios a connection can be recognised between the extremes of transience (unbridled consumerism) and the eternal (totalitarianism), and particular renderings of the relationship between individual and society. The first is of NRT connected to a form of consumerism and consumer choice (for example, conception becomes like 'baby shopping'). Here, NRT is being connected to an extreme example of practices generally current. I interpret this scenario as a particular rendering of the individual/society relationship. In this case, the individual or individualism is predominant and the interpretations of society become less evident, even hidden (cf. Strathern 1992a: 158). The second scenario is of NRT connected to a futuristic vision of the 'Brave New World' or the retrospective one of 'Hitlerism' or the 'master race'. In this set of scenarios, as I interpret them, society is predominant and all powerful (cf. Lefort 1986: 305). This set negates the significance of the individual and individuality (expressed in sentiments such as 'we all become standardised'). Here, the potentials inherent in NRT are extrapolated to a totalitarian vision of future society. The third scenario is evoked in the way NRT belongs to the various techniques by which a heterosexual couple seek to create the child that will be formed through the equal contributions of both the man and woman. I interpret this as making the relationship between individual and society visible, and indeed enabling it in the context of the NRT where otherwise men and women sense its subversion.

My interpretations gather together and make sense of various remarks people made. The third scenario itself brought together the other two. Indeed, the tension between reconciling the desires and choices of the individual with their relationship to society was an explicit and recurring theme in the discussions I held with all of the couples. Each couple, through their own idioms and with reference to their own personal experiences, attempted to sustain a notion of balance and regulation between 'individual' and 'society' made potentially precarious by developments in NRT. I suggest that one means of achieving this, and one evidently available to these couples, was being able to draw on the scenario of conjugality in the context of the NRT: one could improve on 'nature' while remaining true to 'nature's' principles.[2]

THE CONTEXT: THE DIVERSITY OF FAMILIES

The people to whom I spoke (my 'informants') come from a diverse range of family backgrounds, of religious, social and economic circumstances and of educational qualifications. All are involved in conjugal living arrangements. In this sense, conjugality can be taken as a given in informants' circumstances. At the same time, however, there is a diversity in the way each couple has constituted its version of conjugality: remarriage after divorce; foster and/or adopted children present; living close to one 'side' of the family; being distant from both 'sides' of the family, and so forth. As Strathern (1992a: 22) has pointed out:

> While individuals strive to exercise their ingenuity and individuality in the way they create their unique lives, they also remain faithful to a conceptualisation of a natural world as diverse and manifold. Individual partners come together to make [unified] relationships; yet as parents they ought at the same time to stand in an initial condition of natural differentiation from each other. In the relationships they build and elaborate upon, it is important that the prior diversity and individuality of the partners remain.[3]

This point can be illustrated in the following interchanges. Mary and Richard Dobbs have been married for ten years and have three children. They live in a detached, owner-occupied house in Berkshire. Richard works for the police, while Mary works in social services. Both are in their late thirties and both left school at 16. In discussion with Mary and Richard, the conversation became animated when Richard suggested that developments in genetic engineering would enable parents to pick and choose the sort of child they wanted. Mary vigorously resisted his suggestion. Richard argued that parents would want to choose the way a child is genetically built, thus ensuring a 'perfect' child. Although not current practice at the moment, Richard suggested that developments were already going down this road. As he pointed out:

RD: Well we're already doing it, why do you go to all these clinics and the rest of it?

MD: That's to monitor your health throughout your pregnancy.

RD: Your health and who else?

MD: The health of the baby.

RD: What happens if, in the early stages, that baby is mentally ill?

MD: You have the choice of abortion.

RD: Some people take that choice and have an abortion.

MD: And a lot of people don't.

RD: So what they have done, they have picked they don't want that child because it's not perfect . . .

Mary was ready to agree that 'we' [society as embodied in scientists/medicine] are looking for ways of helping people with infertility and of curing disease. She did not agree, however, with Richard's stronger claim that 'we' [society more generally] were 'looking to create the perfect child, the perfect person or perfect race'. To make her point more force-fully, she drew on the memory of discussions from a previous occasion (see below, p. 95) when the issue of home shopping (tele-shopping) was raised. In that discussion, Richard felt that people would gladly welcome these innovations into the home. But as Mary recalled:

MD: [I]t was something that came up when we had our discussions previously that you felt people would rather sit at home and shop, would rather sit at home in front of the television, than go out and shop. But I don't believe that, and I don't think that will ever happen because people will want to go out and shop because the *desire to be with other people is much stronger than using a computer to save them energy*. So I think in the same way that, something has been developed, research and so on and it may be possible to do what Richard has said, to create this perfect being, but I think pressure from society, from people, will say all right you've created that, but we don't actually want that, that's not what we're looking for. [Emphasis added.]

Mary is making a connection between innovations in consumerism and consumer culture with those in NRT. Implicit in her statement is an analogy between home shopping and baby shopping. Mary is not opposed to shopping, but what becomes clear from her discussion with Richard is that shopping is not simply about the easiest mode of access (i.e. through a television/computer screen) to a desired object. It is also about the experience of acquiring the object in the context of other people. In drawing limits around developments of NRT, Mary is drawing on another familiar domain, of consumerism and the consumer culture, to make her point. At the same time, Richard is making comparisons between current practice and the direction in which he perceives the technology to be developing. Like Mary, he is drawing on a particular conception of what motivates people to action and what desired results they aspire towards. In Richard's formulation, 'individualism' is the operative theme, while in Mary's that of 'society' comes to the forefront.

As with the other married couples I spoke to during the research, Mary and Richard have not had direct contact with NRT. At this point, certain general remarks are in order to help contextualise further the material that forms the substance of this chapter.

The couples recruited[4] in the present research formed part of a recently completed study which had been investigating the relationship between family life and the appropriation and use of domestic technology (ESRC-PICT project: Hirsch 1992). My previous research experience with the families had been extensive (based on eight or nine meetings of several hours in each case). The research format used in the two studies was similar: a structured, but open-ended set of questions and discussion themes. The couples had, therefore, a longstanding relationship with myself as ethnographer and with my style of eliciting information. Given the amount of background information held on each family, the present research was based on a single visit to each couple.

My discussions were conducted in the couples' homes with only the husband and wife present. The questions and themes used in the discussions were ordered in such a way as to move from the most immediate and accessible forms of experience to those presumably more distant and less familiar. The themes covered during the discussions were as follows: (a) the family as an idea; (b) children and parents; (c) technologically assisted reproduction (NRT); (d) donation/surrogacy; (e) degrees of acceptable assistance. Each discussion lasted between 2 and $2\frac{1}{2}$ hours and was tape-recorded.

The couples had no problems in talking generally and hypothetically about the themes covered in the discussions. They were not being asked to speak as representatives of, for instance, their class, age group or religious affiliation, though these were all part of their diverse experiences. Rather, the subject of NRT itself offered a perspective from which the couples were able to formulate viewpoints on their own and others' experiences. My intention was to establish a context where informants could talk in the context of one relationship.

The chapter thus highlights the existence of a 'conjugal sub-text' at work in the discussions. By conjugal sub-text I refer to a specific example of a more general process. The specific example follows from the fact that, in the material presented here, the persons are related through a conjugal relationship. The general process is that people act in the context of relationships and in so doing they act with other people in mind. This is the case whether there are other persons physically present or not. Indeed, I suggest that the dialogue these couples sustained with themselves through discussion with me makes evident one dimension of what Alltown people are doing when speaking as individual persons: they exist as individuals within a field of relationships.[5]

As a consequence, the discussions reported here express a particular 'conjugal' perspective on NRT. At one level, I interpret the views being expressed by the couples as related to the way each person understands themselves within their relationship. But, perhaps at a more fundamental level, I infer that the narratives reported here turn on certain axiomatic assumptions about the nature of conjugality itself.[6]

I use the term 'conjugal' rather than 'nuclear' [family] in order to stress the cultural completeness of the husband–wife pair, whether or not the pair is further completed by children (Goody 1983). This accompanies the idea that persons ordinarily have as part of their family experience both a mother and a father. As a norm this is, of course, contested, and is a cultural not a social fact. It is therefore not surprising that the status of the family in English and Western European history is itself a contested issue.[7] Whether we follow Laslett and see the one form as prevailing, or Anderson and see a diverse range, what is clear is that the idea of conjugality strongly impinges upon what is imaginable as 'family life' (cf. Strathern 1992a: 24). To consider the NRT in the context of a conjugal setting is at the same time to conjure up a cultural microcosm informed by ideas intrinsic to English/ Western European kinship thinking. The scenarios that were evoked in discussions with the couples emerged as a way of negotiating limits to what the men and women were prepared to present or express as morally acceptable.

CHILDREN AND PARENTS

Christine Dole of Berkshire heard about the so-called 'virgin birth' controversy when it made its way into the media in 1991. She and her husband
had discussed it at the time and both 'disagreed' with such procedures.
Christine and Daniel have four children; one from her previous marriage,
two from their current marriage. They also have a young adopted son from
an Afro-Caribbean family, whom they had initially fostered. For longer or
shorter periods, there are always one or two foster children in the Dole
home. In fact, both Daniel and Christine would like to make fostering their
full-time occupation, with Daniel leaving his current job (Daniel works for
an international airline; Christine calls herself a housewife). At the moment
they feel they have to add fostering to other activities. The Doles consider
themselves practising Methodists.

CD: I think every child has the right to two parents. If God had wanted us
to have children being only one person we would have been able to
do it. . . . I know a lot of children don't have two parents but a lot of
one parent families do have contact with the other parent.

The practice of egg or sperm donation of itself did not pose a problem for
Christine:

CD: I have no problem with that. If there are reasons why either the man
can't produce the sperm, or the female can't produce the eggs themselves, and they are still a couple and they still want children . . .

Daniel agreed with his wife. But as with a number of other men
and women, he also drew out a darker, more nefarious side to these
processes:

DD: I have a concern, because I think this is where you start to get into
genetic engineering, as far as the people who actually have the money
to select the sperm and/or egg.
CD: Oh no, I wouldn't do it like that, it would have to be, as far as I'm
concerned, I think sperm and eggs should be labelled white or black
or mixed race and that's as far as it should go.

But Daniel still felt there was a more powerful side to the technologies that
could not be controlled:

DD: I feel pretty certain that things are going to get pretty muddled and perhaps that's why certain people are beginning to say No, the white race must be there, or No, we must have this or No, we must have that . . . perhaps that's what's actually prompting some of the work that's actually done, because there are people in power, in authority who are able to promote these things and pay for them to actually occur, who could perhaps be engineering this super race.

Daniel felt that the women wanting a 'virgin birth' should be counselled. He felt there were many children already born that needed adoptive parents. Christine agreed. For her, couples have children and if a single person wants a child, they should be able to adopt. This would allow, in her view, a deeper 'truth' to be revealed.

CD: [B]y saying they want to adopt they will then have lots of counselling and their reasons for wanting a child so desperately as a single person would be gone into properly.

Underlying the concerns of both Christine and Daniel were the issues of keeping certain facts or tendencies outside of the context of having children (for example, money, anonymous donating third parties and totalitarian power). It is for these reasons they found adoption and even surrogacy, if money did not change hands, such suitable alternatives.

CD: [I]n which case, if there's no money changing hands and the surrogate had nothing to do with either parent, then basically what we're saying is that the surrogate mother gives the baby up for adoption and the couple adopt it and then in that case I don't think it makes any difference at all.

If these elements entered into the context of the child's life, certain problems would become manifest:

DD: . . . whether the child is actually at some stage in the future going to have an identity crisis, going to wonder about the other party, that wasn't involved . . . in their upbringing and all the rest of it.

I suggest that what the Doles (and other couples) are seeking to maintain is the idea that parents should reproduce persons who are individuals in themselves: 'that individual persons are somehow prior to . . . relationship', one of Strathern's facts of English kinship (1992a: 53; see n. 3 above). The introduction of these other elements into the situation of a child's 'individuality' is seen potentially to subvert this process; the child's 'individuality' is evidently being formed through various public and visible relationships instead of existing prior to them.

Like the Doles, Ganesh and Rajni Lunn, who live in a Westminster owner-occupied maisonette with their three daughters, had followed the item in the tabloids at the time. Ganesh and Rajni came to London from South Africa nearly twenty years ago, but their families originate from India. Their links to Hinduism are explicit in their home, with daily prayers, especially on Friday evenings. Ganesh is often called to act as priest for family ceremonies. They refer to themselves as a 'modern' family and, after so long in Britain, think of themselves as having taken on many of the attitudes associated with British family life. But this form of conception went too far.

RL: We felt it wasn't right for a woman to have a test tube baby without having any sexual connections with a male . . .

GL: What kind of feeling would she have, she's nothing else than a factory, like a conveyor belt conveying the completed product . . .

And in developing these ideas he adds:

GL: Yes, it's the vision Hitler had of a superhuman race, isn't it. . . . It's contrary and contradictory to the role of Nature isn't it, where you are now propagating the role of Nature.

Both Rajni and Ganesh appear to be strongly opposed to forms of NRT. Their objections, however, are less focused on the techniques themselves than on the consequences for relations between parent and child. This emerged in more explicit fashion later in our discussions when we considered the possibilities of multiple births under certain NRT procedures. As Rajni indicates, she is not against multiple births *per se*:

RL: [It's O]kay, right, for example say a man and woman can't get together to fertilise and have babies, and the eggs are taken out from her and the sperm is taken from the man and are fertilised outside and then put back into the woman, it's still the same man and woman who's doing it, for me that's okay, it doesn't matter how many multiple births you have, it's still the same man and same woman who have produced it. The problem arises for me when there's man and woman and they have to bring a third party in to create that from the sperm bank, that worries me because then what do you tell the child where it originally comes from, or who the father is?

The problem for Rajni, as well as her husband, was the existence of a third party outside the original mother and father pair. In pushing her point forward, she draws on the now well-established and familiar cultural icon of Louise Brown (see Chapter 1).[8]

RL: Because when you look at our test tube, how old is she?

EH: Who's this, Louise Brown?

RL: Yes, but in her case it's her mother and father, it's not brought from outside, there's no third party involved, it's just its own natural mother and father, it was only fertilised outside and put into a test tube. That's Okay because she knows that is her natural father although she's been brought into this world in a different way from other children.

As in the case of the Doles, adoption was seen by Rajni and Ganesh as a preferable alternative. Although the adopted child would have the trauma of its early life outside a family to contend with, through the adoptive process this would be transformed. Ganesh felt that gradually this early emotional state would 'wear' away. He contrasted this process with that of surrogacy and, in particular, surrogacy where there was a transaction of money. Again, the image of a consumer process was evoked to characterise the negative aspects of this relationship with a child:

GL: [I]t's like going into a supermarket and taking a baby off the shelf, putting it in the trolley, wheeling it to the cashier, paying the cashier and walking off with the child. It's not that simple.

Again, the question of the child's identity became the issue. Rajni returned to the example of Louise Brown. Although she was seen to exemplify the positive side of NRT, the way she came into the world raised problems of identity and difference. Rajni wondered whether the circumstances of her birth and the large media attention in subsequent years would cause her to become 'anti-people'; or whether people will become 'anti-towards-her'. These are all factors she will have to cope with, while, as Rajni pointed out, her children will not have to cope with such problems.[9]

Whereas in their particular ways Christine and Daniel, like Rajni and Ganesh, were in general agreement about these issues, Megan and Nicholas Selby had very different perspectives from each other. Megan and Nicholas live in a council flat in Camden with their two sons. Megan is a part-time play instructor for the local council; Nicholas works in a small local travel agency. Megan knew they would disagree when we began to discuss the issues touched on by the research. She said the two of them had very different opinions about 'equal ops and that sort of subject'.

MS: I honestly don't see why they ['virgin birth women'] can't just go to a sperm bank, I don't want a relationship, I might be gay, I might be whatever you want to call it, lesbian, I want to have a child anyway.

Although she saw single women conceiving through artificial means as acceptable, Megan was not in favour of what she called 'cloning'; this is where she drew the limit. As she put it:

MS: Sperm bank babies, and they can choose what colour hair, skin, mentality depending on whose sperm it is . . . it's a type of cloning.

By contrast, Nicholas had a great difficulty in initially accommodating any aspect of these forms of reproduction.

NS: It's not a natural relationship, it's not a relationship that's natural to have children, two females or for that matter two males, cannot produce children.

Nicholas's expressed concern was in relation to the child.

NS: I don't think it's fair on the child.
MS: What's not fair?
NS: Because that child will not have a 'normal' relationship.
MS: But it would be [normal] to that child but not to you.
NS: Nor to anybody else. It's an abnormal relationship.

On this point there was no agreement between Megan and Nicholas. From Megan's earlier comments, they had certainly disagreed on this and similar issues in the past. Where they did agree was around what Megan had referred to as 'cloning', and more specifically on the use of genetic engineering to produce a particular sort of child. To elaborate her point, Megan drew on her own relationship with Nicholas; there was a virtue for society at large in the way they had paired up.

MS: This is where people like Nicholas and I for some unknown reason attract, it brings things into a norm. I'm so short and he's tall, and it brings the offspring to a middling size, so their offspring should continue a natural balance, and I think that if you start messing about with the genetics until . . .
NS: In its place it's fine [egg and sperm donation], if it can help a couple who want children, who can't have children naturally, to have children, great, but if it comes to the state where you're messing around

with genetics to produce, you're getting back into almost the realms of the Aryan race. You're trying to create something to an ideal.

The disagreements between Megan and Nicholas stemmed from different versions of what they imagined was 'natural' or normal and what was 'unnatural'. On further reflection, and after listening to Megan's comments, Nicholas felt he was able to accommodate a particular image of NRT:

NS: If you can give a couple, who want children, the ability to have children by artificial insemination by fertilising the egg inside, outside the body whatever then reimplanting, fine, you're giving Nature a helping hand. But if you're trying to create the master race, by fiddling around with genetics, that's wrong.

I suggest that as long as the image of a man and woman contributing equally to the child was sustained, Nicholas could imagine the acceptability of these techniques. If this type of assistance did not bring the desired result, then (Nicholas insisted) the only alternative was adoption. Although the child was not the 'flesh and blood' of either parent, each could feel they were equally contributing to it as a parent. He was insistent that if the child had the genetic substance of only one parent, then the relationship between the parents would not work.

NS: Then it wouldn't last, if you've got such a, if the woman really so desperately wants children that badly, every argument you get, that you have, that will keep being thrown backwards and forwards and in the end that relationship wouldn't last.

PERSPECTIVES ON CONNECTEDNESS

We have just seen how couples from diverse family contexts approach the image of a single mother wanting to conceive a child without a male partner present. In each case, they negotiated possibilities and drew limits around what they were prepared to present as morally acceptable. Their thoughts were constrained by contrary images of consumerism, totalitarianism and the loss of individuality, and by the apparent desire to keep a 'natural' relationship between the individual and society through conjugality. This is true despite the way the arguments vary. Megan Selby, for example, is prepared to allow the 'virgin birth' as acceptable; she at the same time draws limits around what she will not condone ('cloning'). When I raised similar questions, not in relation to a distant and hypothetical other (virgin mother), but in relation to one's own reproductive substance (donation), I found men and women drawing similar conclusions – though in the course of doing so they might use different images to evoke the same three scenarios.

Natalie and Charles Simon live in a large terraced house in Islington. They have five children, two of whom are adopted. Natalie is a part-time teacher and Charles describes himself as a technologist or inventor. They also have a summer house and boat on the south-west coast.

When I discussed egg and sperm donation with them, Charles indicated he would not do this; it would be beyond any limit he was prepared to go to: 'I wouldn't be prepared to put all the other resources . . . donating the physical genes that's not the problem is it, as I see it?' Charles then elaborated on the idea:

CS: I wouldn't be prepared to donate sperm because I couldn't back it up with the emotional support, all the other support that I think as a result of that donation would require. I would feel obliged to not donate a sperm but donate the whole package, the responsibility of it.

Natalie agreed in absolute terms with her husband. For both, the idea of donation evoked the image of parenthood and one could not be dissociated from the other.

Earlier in our discussion, Natalie and Charles spoke of their family life as a 'project' [their term]. They conceptualised its organisation in this manner: initially certain things had to be put into place (finances, a place to live). Charles also indicated that the 'project' is periodically 'reviewed'; they discuss and plan what they are going to do in the future and when it will happen. When they got married, the intention was to have children; it was some years before this actually happened, but as Charles put it, 'it was always on the agenda'. Neither of them could imagine the disassociation of this project from their own genetic substance – the one was part of the other. In fact, during the years leading up to having their first child, they had explicitly considered the possibilities of infertility and adoption: these were options they felt needed to be considered as part of the process of carrying out their project. As it turned out, they decided to adopt in any case.

The donation of genetic substance raised the issue of the lengths to which men and women were prepared to go in order to have a child. Natalie felt uncomfortable with certain practices. She brought into the discussion the example of a friend who was unable to have children with her husband.

NS: I have a friend who's married, her husband was infertile, she desperately wanted a child, so she had an affair with somebody else and got
pregnant and had a child. As the child is growing up, she has told the
child that her husband was not his natural father, but the child, I
think, is incredibly confused about the relationship, he knows his
mother had an affair with this other person, and he knows this other
person, and if you know who donated the sperm or eggs, I think in
some ways that is going to affect your relationship later on.

Charles felt that in such a situation the child was being put in the position of
a 'freak': 'It has an identity of itself as something radically different and
unusual from its peers.' The only context in which he could imagine the
acceptability of such practices (including NRT) was one of what he called
'alternative parenthood'.

CS: I can see it would work in a situation where you had an extended
family, that you were living in an environment where several couples,
with their parents and their children were all mixed up. . . . Where a
group of adults took on the collective role of parents to a group of
children. . . . And if they went outside that environment they would
have the resources, they would have the assistance of the group that
they were brought up with, and they could get support . . . self-
identity in that way.

Both Natalie and Charles agreed that the identity of the child could be
adversely affected by the various techniques of donation and assistance now
possible with NRT. What was of most concern to both was the tendency
to transform the basis of childhood itself. In their view, the parent has a
'mission' to help the child become a 'happy and integrated member of
society'. In the context of NRT, there is a tendency to end up with a
different type of child:

CS: [T]herefore you end up with a different type of child; *its mind will
have been formed by relationships which are different from a child that
was created by other means.* [Emphasis added.]

When I discussed gamete donation with Eileen and Phil O'Leary, a different set of connections were evoked. The O'Learys live in a semi-detached
house in Berkshire with their four children. Their eldest son is currently
sitting his A-levels and plans to attend university next year. Eileen has been a
housewife most of her married life but has recently started working in social
services; Phil started his own business during the late 1980s after working

for over a decade in a large London department store. They were both raised as Catholics, although Phil now considers himself an agnostic.

EH: Would you be prepared to be a donor with your sperm?
PO: I haven't got any now, it's irrelevant.
EH: Oh, you've had a vasectomy?
PO: Yes.
EH: But assuming . . .
PO: I think I would have.
EO: Now, I wouldn't let Phil do that willingly, now you said you wouldn't mind, I would actually give that some thought, that sounds really selfish doesn't it? I was quite possessive then!

And a short while later Eileen expands on her initial reaction.

EO: It was almost like he was being unfaithful, the initial feeling was Oh, he was being a bit free and easy . . .

In this context, Phil indicated that by donating sperm he would be doing his 'bit for society', but for Eileen the thought evoked an initial reaction of unfaithfulness. It was as if Phil were prepared to commit adultery: to behave in a very individual and selfish way. The initial contrast between Eileen and Phil's attitude in this context bears comparison with Megan and Nicholas Selby in the last section. It will be recalled that Megan was prepared to accept a number of innovations associated with the NRT that Nicholas found unacceptable. In the present couple, Eileen appears to adopt a more conservative perspective than her husband.[10]

EO: [I don't agree] that a single parent should automatically be able to go to a sperm bank and have their eggs fertilised . . . it's a dodgy business for later on in life for that particular child.

Again, Eileen's reflections on techniques of donation lead her to consider the possible effects it has on the child's mind: 'It just sounds awful coming from a sperm, coming from a freezer.' Phil, by contrast, has a more accepting, if slightly cynical, attitude towards these developments. On the one hand, he finds it difficult to separate these techniques from other controversial research in science and its technological implementation.

PO: And you really can't differentiate between biological experimentation like that and filling the world with nuclear arms, because it's the very same thing, science is following research as far as it will go.

But this view is wedded to one which senses an inevitability to these trends, and their negative if somewhat desired outcomes.

PO: When you get into it, the very fact that it's done, for instance, if somebody goes to a sperm bank, somebody goes to a baby shop to get a baby ... what I'm saying is look at the lovely guarantees you've got, it won't be abnormal because they've screened the embryo to make sure there's nothing wrong with it, before it's implanted ... it's not Nature's work any more. It's somebody getting a microscope and saying Oh, don't like that one, that one's not perfect, get rid of that one, or people saying, I'm not having that embryo it's a girl. Then you can literally end up going shopping for a baby.

Whereas Eileen felt the sense of adultery and betrayal by Phil's casual offer to donate sperm, Phil sensed a certain inevitability associated with developments in NRT which led to a close connection between babies and consumerism. Neither Eileen nor Phil thought NRT should be abandoned. Rather they suggested that NRT presented the possibility of novel forms of relationships (particularly linked to anonymous donation) which challenged our existing morals. The image of a child as the product of two known parents was at the centre of their conceptions.

In discussion with a London-based couple, Lynn and Frank Irving, an analogous reference was made to adultery. Lynn and Frank live in a council flat in Camden with their daughter and son. Frank sells insurance while Lynn describes herself as a housewife, but also does voluntary work at their son's school. Both are Jewish. I asked Lynn her thoughts about human egg and sperm donation:

LI: At one stage I used to think yes, it was nothing, I hadn't really thought about it and even suggested to a friend of mine ...
EH: What did you suggest?
LI: That she should have artificial insemination.

At this point the husband, Frank immediately added, 'Test tube adultery'.

Eileen's response focused on unfaithfulness with an anonymous other; Lynn's advice to a friend to seek an anonymous donor suggested to Frank adultery, albeit in a test tube. By none of these three couples could sperm be imagined as an entity divorced from various social/sexual relationships; even Phil's donation to 'society' led to an image, given voice by his wife, of potential illicit sex. Lynn then went on to add:

LI: But then, thinking about it years later, I don't think it's a good idea. I think it comes to a point in one's life where you have to accept your limitations, and if you really can't have a child from your partner, and it's absolutely impossible, if you can't adopt a child . . . and if there isn't a child to adopt, well I think one has to accept their limitations.

Lynn argued that when one was able to face up to these limitations, the next possible option was to consider adopting a child. We also discussed the fact that the number of children available for adoption was in relative terms not very large. Even so, they both insisted that an anonymous donation was unacceptable. If NRT had to be brought into the process, then it should only involve the substance of the husband and wife.

LI: I don't object to fertilisation within the test tube, with a husband and wife's fertilisation . . .

FI: [I]t keeps it within its own context both genetically, biologically and psychologically, they say it is us, it needed some artificial assistance, but it's us that actually produced it, it's our baby, it's not 50 per cent somebody else.

Earlier in our discussion, Lynn and Frank described to me the way they felt connected to their children. As in the case of many of the couples, they did not mention a genetic connection (it was ideas of love, responsibility, support, respect and so on that were usually mentioned).

EH: But before, when we were talking about the way you felt you were connected to your children . . . you didn't really mention that at all.

FI: But you take it for granted. It's only when you're suddenly confronted with the possibility it could not be your child.

Lynn then suggested the following analogy:

LI: Look, imagine [a roof] and you're holding it up with [two] pillar[s], those pillars are not joined together, they are apart, they are standing apart, but they are still part of each other because they have one aim to hold that roof up, as one pillar collapses, then the other can't support that beam, so even though they are separate, they are still one, so are children. Even though you're separate, you are still one, do you understand what I'm getting at? But you cannot think of that child all the time as an extension of yourself, an extension of your character, of everything within yourself, they are a separate individual but they are still part of you.

As we have seen in other conjugal contexts, what one reproduces as a parent is a separate yet 'connected' individual. Both Lynn and Frank are suggesting that the advent of the NRT brings the potential for those ideas of love, responsibility and so forth, that are explicitly associated with (parents) being connected to a child, as becoming 'disconnected' from their previously implicit foundation in a genetic base.

Unlike Lynn, though, Mark Lyon did not give advice to a friend to seek an anonymous donation. But, as with Lynn Irving, his perception of these matters changed over time. Mark and his wife Shirley of Berkshire live in an owner-occupied semi-detached house. They have three daughters and one son. The eldest daughter has recently completed secondary school. Shirley works as a director's personal assistant in a computer firm; Mark has a middle-management position in a multi-national technology company. They fostered children in the past, before the birth of their first child.

Mark explained his change of attitude as being linked to an article he had read.

ML: I used to think this was fairly socially acceptable, the act of sperm donation, medical students of the 1960s used to do this to earn some extra money to pay their way through college, they used to donate sperm and this was used in AID [artificial insemination by donor]. . . . But then I actually read, a couple of years ago, some references to people who had grown up and had discovered that this was how they had come into the world. Now this was about the time that adopted children in this country were given freer access to their original birth certificates. . . . At the same time, a story surfaced from people who were products of insemination by donor and it was really quite revealing, it took me aback, in that these people were actually angry with their sperm father, as they called it, because they said, What sort of careless thing to do, to go in, to donate sperm, walk away with some money, and not give another thought to what was to follow on from that, to never know the consequences of that.

Shirley Lyon shared her husband's feelings on this issue.

SL: I think it's sad in the case of the people who've grown up and discovered that the person you think is your natural father isn't . . . and the fact that the husband, father, that must be quite something to accept the fact that your wife's going to have a baby but genetically it's not yours . . .

Mark and Shirley both stressed the potential unhappiness created by the techniques of sperm donation. On the one hand, the child may discover (or in fact be told) that they came into the world as a result of another person's genetic material. On the other hand, the husband, for example, may have to live with the fact that the child he loves and values is 'not really his'. In the light of the difficulties associated with such artificial techniques, I suggested to Mark and Shirley that perhaps they should be discontinued. Although they both acknowledged that numerous problems, both inter- and intra-personal, resulted from the use of the techniques, neither of them suggested that the techniques should no longer be available.

SL: No, because I don't think everybody that happens to, I mean when you have a child, even if it isn't [yours], when you raise a child from a baby, and you've loved it and cared for it, you taught it all the things that you value and you hope that it will grow up to be a confident human being, then I feel that it does, that child is part of you whether or not you made it in the first place.

Shirley was insistent that if the parents had considered the situation with a great amount of thought and discussion, and had prepared themselves for all the later consequences, then they should be fine. But she added that it took a special sort of person (especially on the part of the 'father' or 'mother') to be able to bring a child into the world in this way.

We continued this line of discussion for some time, after which I asked Shirley and Mark whether they thought such donations should be from a known person or should be anonymous. Mark suggested that with an anonymous donor the whole process might be easier to accept. He said that one heard stories about those who choose traits they desired in the child, even though the donor was anonymous. Mark's comments sparked a con- nection in Shirley's mind. She was immediately reminded of a conversation she had with a neighbour a few years before. Her recollection of this con- versation also connected with her earlier comments on techniques of sperm and egg donation. Although a potential source of sadness and confusion for all parties concerned, such techniques, she felt, should not be discontinued: if the child is given enough love and care they will 'be a part of you whether or not you made the child in the first place'.

SL: What Mark said before, took me back, just a flash in my mind, to a conversation I had with a . . . next-door neighbour of mine . . . and her sister had been adopted. Now I didn't know that because those two girls looked so much alike I would never had known that they weren't natural sisters. . . . We had a conversation about it and they said we guess we just grew alike, it was so strange.

I asked Shirley why this *particular* recollection was brought to mind.

SL: This business of saying, Well I'd like to have the donor who donated the sperm, if he could have blue eyes and brown hair or whatever, a ginger moustache. . . . Maybe when people are living close together, they do look alike, maybe it's the way they cut their hair, or their facial expressions or the way they stand, I don't know.

Mark then succinctly elaborated on Shirley's insight.

ML: Your expectations, so you expect it, *you see what you want to see . . .* [Emphasis added.]

DIFFERENCES OF OPINION

How one perceives a child born under circumstances of donation and/or surrogacy became a point of disagreement in my discussions with the Dobbses. It will also be recalled from earlier in this chapter that Mary and Richard had different perspectives on the long-term possibilities made available by developments in genetic engineering: Richard suggested that parents might be attracted by the possibility of genetically producing a perfect child, while Mary argued that, although this might be technically possible, it was not what people generally wanted.

It emerged during the course of our conversation that Mary had considered, at some point in the past, being a surrogate mother for her sister. Her sister had had a miscarriage and the medical diagnosis given afterwards seemed to suggest that she suffered from a rare disorder which might prevent her from giving birth to children (it subsequently transpired that she was able to have children and now has two). Mary said she cared very much for her sister and knew the sort of feelings that exist when one wants to have a baby. At the time, Mary discussed the possibility of acting as a surrogate first with her sister and then separately with Richard. The conversations were recalled by Richard and he said that his views had not changed since that time. In essence, he was not in favour of Mary acting as a surrogate for her sister:

RD: Mary's my wife, Mary has my children, not somebody else's.

Richard said that he would feel alienated from this child, knowing that it was a part of Mary and had nothing to do with him. When Mary asked him to think about the *reasons* she had for considering to take on this role, Richard replied:

RD: I hear what you're saying, very commendable, but at the end of the day you and I are number one and it is us we should think about.

What underlined these differences were opposing attitudes to the intentions behind donation itself. Richard felt it should be given and received anonymously, while Mary said she would want to know whom her eggs were being used to help; she would want the recipient to know her.

MD: I would like to know who I am donating it to and why.
RD: You don't think you'd have feelings for that kid when it's born?
MD: No, I don't think I would, I might have a closer relationship possibly, but I can't speculate on that, but I wouldn't be doing it for that reason, the overriding feeling would be . . .
RD: You've just hit a point there, a closer relationship with that child.
MD: I don't know, but one can't always view things from one's own perspective can one, one has to look at things from other people's point of view.

Much of the subsequent discussion revolved around how one would 'look' at a child that was a product of the donation of either sperm or egg.

RD: I'd see him every birthday, christening, you know what I mean, and I think if it was my child, I think every time I saw that child one thing that would go through my mind.

Mary then directed our attention to the fact that we had failed to consider the perspective of the child in these matters.

MD: The one person we haven't actually talked about is the child and their feelings at the end of the day, and how would that child feel, growing up and it might be that Mum says well I want to tell you this because I want to be truthful to you about you and where you come from but Richard is really your dad.

Although Mary did not initially consider this to be an important consideration – from her adult perspective – when she began to view matters from the perspective of the child, many more complications emerged than first seemed to appear. Richard suggested that such information might come out into the open, given certain circumstances, and be used in a hurtful manner.

RD: All it needs is an upset in the family, you could turn round and say that child is mine, all sorts of nasty things could come out, like the father could not produce the child, it's not my child, we don't know who the father is because it's all anonymous.

The Dobbses perceived numerous tensions and potential conflicts arising from new forms of reproduction and the technologies associated with them. A number of the issues they raised in their discussion, particularly the distinction between 'a father' and 'a real [in their view, genetic] father', are not necessarily confined to developments associated with NRT. On both points, there is an overlap between the discussion I had with the Dobbses and that with the Murphys, although this latter couple came to the discussion from a particular family background.

Winnie and Ted Murphy live in Berkshire. They have an owner-occupied semi-detached house and share it with one of the two children from Ted's previous marriage. They also own a caravan in south-west England. Both Winnie and Ted have been married previously. They have been in their present marriage for six years. Ted is in his mid-fifties and has recently taken early retirement from his job as a trade-union official; Winnie is a nurse and recently completed a university degree. The eldest child, Caroline, started a course at university last year, while Sam is studying for his state exams (A-levels) and still lives at home.

The tensions that were expressed by the Dobbses – especially around the 'unequal' contribution to a child's birth (whether genetically or through gestation) – also became evident when Winnie and Ted discussed the same set of issues. In this case, however, they emerged from a baseline different from that of the other families. During the early part of our discussion, Winnie and Ted were asked to offer some thoughts about their family. As with the other couples, a distinction was soon introduced between immediate or close family and relatives (cf. Firth *et al.* 1969: 89–98). Winnie spoke of immediate family as being about close contact, the people we know better than others, as compared to relatives who are more distant. But Ted soon introduced a further distinction which seemed to complicate matters:

TM: It is more than closeness. . . . Immediate family would include my mother and father because we are part of them. From them we have been created and my brothers share that creation because they come from the same womb, so I would see that as immediate family. I see our children as being immediate family because they are from our creation. But your aunts and uncles haven't got that kind of relationship.

Ted's attempt to encompass both their thoughts with this comment contradicted a fundamental aspect of his conjugal experience with Winnie: namely, 'their' children were not a product of their 'creation'. Winnie soon put another gloss on his remark.

WM: I don't know that I necessarily see it like that, I think it's more to do with closeness you have with certain members of the family.

She then expanded on this point:

WM: Well, how much you sort of share with them, like although I won't see my sister's baby a lot, not closeness in the sense that you see them a lot, but I speak to them a lot, we share all sorts of childhood experiences and things like that. I don't know whether it's necessarily simply just coming from the same womb, because I see Caroline and Sam as my kids, but they're not, do you know what I mean? But they are still classed as family.

The implicit tension between a 'biological/natural' connection with the children and a 'social' connection was a recurring theme throughout our conversation. At several points, Winnie stressed that although Caroline and Sam were not her biological children, Caroline, in particular, considers her to be the mother: 'Mothering has been me, she sees that as me.' Ted agreed with Winnie on these points throughout the discussion. However, it was his periodic recourse to a conception of parenthood based on 'biological' facts which frequently necessitated Winnie to stress the non-biological dimension of parenting. For example, I asked them to consider those factors which could prevent one from being a parent. Ted immediately started to answer but was cut short by Winnie:

TM: Apart from biological things . . .
WM: I don't think that's true because we've just said all that. I'm parenting although I'm not the biological mother, that's nothing to do with it.

Again, after we had covered the topics of donation and technologically assisted forms of reproduction, this same tension emerged later with respect to dimensions of maternal surrogacy. Both Winnie and Ted agreed that people should seek out adoption – trying to give a home to children who have no parents – as opposed to choosing artificial means of bringing a child into the world. But Ted suggested there was a thin line dividing adoption and surrogacy: in a surrogate birth, the child has to be signed over by the biological mother and in this way there is little technical difference between it and adoption. He then went on to make an additional point:

TM: I don't know, but I would find it very difficult to come to terms with, as the child is growing up, to see the features of the mother, appearing in the child, and they're not your features.[11]

Ted's comment was again unsettling for Winnie, particularly as her relationship with Caroline and Sam seemed to replicate the difficulty he had identified for himself. To distinguish her own experience from these other forms of parenting, Winnie brought into the discussion what she called the 'cultural inheritance': the 'cultural thing' one passes on to one another. She was not able to elaborate on this idea, but it was clear she was making a distinction between what one acquires through culture, and what in this case she called a 'nurturing [biological] mother'. But again, this holds as true for adoption and being a stepmother. In order to overcome the dilemma and distinguish surrogacy from the experience of Winnie *vis-à-vis* the children, Ted stated that surrogacy arrangements are tainted by a commercial attitude:

TM: They see children as a market . . .
WM: Just another commodity to be bought and sold on an open market.

This agreement signalled a joint perspective. Both step-parenthood and adoption could be seen to be sustaining the link, however partially, between the 'natural' and 'social': what they share is the way they keep relationships separate from aspects of money and the market.

Markets, materialism and morality

Winnie and Ted, as with the other couples I spoke to, attached negative consequences to developments in NRT. Reference to Brave New World and Hitlerism emerged time and again during our talks. This totalitarian scenario was evoked precisely when the possibilities of choice and selection were made apparent by the techniques associated with NRT: the idea that one could now select and construct 'the perfect race'. In fact, Winnie even suggested that if we lived in a different, perhaps non-capitalistic society, these same fears would not be evident. However, given the world we live in, one cannot but feel that it 'has sinister implications'.

Some of these same concerns were expressed by Gloria and Paul De Guy, also of Berkshire. But the conjugal context from which they were expressing their views was very different from that just considered. Gloria and Paul live in an owner-occupied detached house with three young children. Gloria calls herself a housewife and Paul works in a management capacity for a large telecommunications company. They both consider themselves devout Catholics and their Catholic beliefs impinged strongly during our discussion.[12] In fact, I attempted to discuss several of the themes associated with donation, surrogacy and NRT, themes I explored with the other couples, but the conversations were curtailed very quickly: Gloria and Paul were totally 'against' them as a matter of religious principles. They discussed the possibilities only long enough to register their disagreement. Gloria summed up her thoughts in the following way:

GD: I, myself, am torn in two, I find it very hard, on the one hand a part of me believes that yes, you have to use whatever knowledge and intellect you have to solve all manner of human problems and one of them would be infertility. However, having said that, I think infertility would be very low down my scale of priorities of helping the human race, in that particular situation it's a question of God's will. If you're meant to have them, you will and it is unreasonable in my mind to go to the lengths that apparently one has to conceive a child.

Gloria, in particular, saw developments in NRT as part of a wider trend in society. She did not see NRT as an innovation that came about and then had effects on the attitudes of people (as suggested by comments of other people I spoke to). Rather, it reflected a selfishness that was intrinsic to society and allowed people to expand the areas where they could be selfish.

GD: It's yet another way of getting round life, of doing what they want to do, putting themselves, their own needs absolutely first: I want a baby, I'm upset, I'm going to do whatever it takes to do it, like I want a car, I'll go and get a bank loan and I'll get a car. It's like another possession, another thing they want and they will move heaven and earth to get it.

It is the image of unbridled consumerism that Gloria and, to a lesser extent, Paul picked up on: 'a danger of seeing [a baby] as yet another material possession'. She perceived a trend where children just become the next thing in the long list of material possessions one is supposed to have. This is the process Gloria sees at work in relation to NRT.

GD: I don't for a moment wish to be unkind to the couples who genuinely are bitterly disappointed and would love to have it for the right reasons, but for many it isn't that, it's like you get a car, a dishwasher and then a dog and then you think what next . . . so I think there is that sort of danger to it, that one perceives them as the thing to have, the thing to do.

For Gloria and Paul, if children come 'naturally' within the married state, then this was another matter altogether. All attempts artificially to assist the process were wrong. Gloria put it in strong terms: 'I feel that the whole field of procreation ought to be left alone.'

These same issues were not so clear-cut for Maria and Geoff Williams. Both are trained pharmacists and work in two of the local hospitals. They have a daughter and son and live in a semi-detached, owner-occupied house in Berkshire. When we began to touch on some of the issues described for the De Guys, Geoff indicated that such matters had been familiar to them for a long time, given their medical background and working environment. Maria supported his comments by referring to Louise Brown and the relatively long period that has elapsed since her birth. Geoff was even prepared to suggest that these matters were an 'accepted fact'. Maria was not prepared to go quite so far. She perceived a worrying side to these developments which could not just be glossed over. In particular, she drew on the image of genetic engineering and, more specifically, the possibility that men and women will be able to decide in the future what sort of child they want. This is a suggestion we have come across in various ways already. Geoff concurred with Maria, while at the same time arguing that all of these developments would have to occur under strict controls. For her, it was the danger of 'it being completely taken over by science'.

Geoff stated it from a different perspective. For him, the advent of trust hospitals in the NHS meant that the market mechanism could be used to provide men and women with these 'services' if they so desired. It would be a matter of supplying people with what they want. His half-joking manner was offset by his experience of 'market forces' having been introduced into his own sector of the hospital:

GW: A trust hospital might go for something like 'special offer this week – red-headed boys'.

For Maria, it all 'smacked of the Aryan race'. Geoff felt less threatened:

GW: It would be possible from a scientific point of view. Lots of things are possible now, it's just they wouldn't morally be accepted.

While Maria was most concerned with the potential 'standardisation' of children in the context of the NRT, Geoff could imagine the potential of innovative hospitals and maternity wards operating in a new market-led environment.

GW: Which comedian was it, Leslie Crowther wasn't it? He had a girl, and another girl, how many girls did he have, four or five girls, what he would have done for a boy, everything except have a sixth girl. Now if he was put in a position where he could have said, If we do this, you'll definitely have a boy, who's to say he wouldn't have gone for it? Who's to say that if we had Ellen and then we'd had another daughter, and I'd say Oh I want a son, if that had been available, say Okay we'll do this and we'll definitely have a boy, that we wouldn't have gone for it?

MW: But I think we would have been prepared to accept that we were going to have another child, and if the child was a girl it would still be our child.

But as Geoff readily acknowledged, all of the developments would be constrained by the current morality and what people thought was morally acceptable. Maria was less convinced by the effectiveness of controls:

MW: It's difficult to say what the point is though, isn't it? Because what would be sound now, in ten years' time, the improvements in science and the improvements in technology, who's to say the barriers won't move?

The problem of morality and its change over time was also a theme that Denis White highlighted towards the end of our discussion. Denis and Margaret live in an owner-occupied semi-detached house in Berkshire with their four young children. Denis works for the Post Office; Margaret describes herself as a housewife and also does some paid child-minding.

Margaret made it clear towards the beginning of our discussion how important children were to her. It was a topic she discussed with Denis before they got married; she did not see any point in getting married to someone who did not want children. Although they never considered adopting children, it was an option that would have arisen very quickly:

MW: I mean obviously if we couldn't have had any, then I would have gone anywhere to find out how I could get them.

During the course of our conversation, Denis and Margaret drew on scenarios that were evoked by several of the other couples. They made connections between techniques of sperm and egg donation with images of catalogue shopping, genetic engineering and 'the master race'. At the same time, they both agreed that a 'conventional' couple (husband and wife) should be given 'all the help that medical science can give them': an image of 50 per cent, or equal shares coming from each partner in a relationship, was their underlying model (they also extended this idea to an adopted child where each can give equal shares, as well as a test-tube baby, where equal shares of substance could be given). Again, as with many of the couples, neither Mary nor Denis had explicitly considered all of the themes and their variations before I raised them during our conversations. It is in this light that Denis made the following observation towards the end of our discussion:

DW: A lot of it really is to say, through these questions, are people's morals or understanding keeping up with the changes in medicine and you know, do people feel all these changes are for the good and are we ready for them? Medicine is racing well ahead; do we morally feel we are in agreement with what they're doing? We probably need time to catch up with the medical people where things will change over the years. *I suppose, given enough time, we will all start to think differently.* [Emphasis added.]

The problem for Denis, as well as several other of the men and women who raised this same possibility, was that no matter how hard these developments are thought about, discussed and even resisted, given enough time, they would change what we are prepared to imagine as thinkable and acceptable. There is a certain inevitability attached to the future that is supposed for such ideas and one that makes change almost inescapable.

CONCLUSION: WHAT KIND OF LIMITS?

Throughout the discussions I had with the couples reported in the pages above, concern was expressed that the way we conduct our most familiar relationships would change dramatically with the advent and greater use of the NRT. Two recurrent scenarios were evoked to express concern, even fear, about how NRT should be appropriated.[13] Each contained images of limits, though the particular images on which people drew were as diverse as their experiences. Then again, concern was expressed that NRT could lead to children being just another aspect of the individualist, consumer culture, so that conception would be reduced to just another feature of shopping and consumption. On the other hand, couples were concerned by the possibility inherent, as they saw it, in NRT producing a master race, where the powerful are in such a strong position that they are able to impose what their vision of society should look like in the future. In either case, the modernist relationship between 'individual' and 'society' is potentially subverted. As one might expect in conversations with people in the context of conjugal relationships, their stated imaginings of how NRT should be appropriated also had a particular conjugal bias. The third scenario offered hope through regulation. NRT should be appropriated so as to sustain the image of a child as a product of a known and present mother and father.

The idioms, however, that the couples use to negotiate their concerns are drawn from domains we would not ordinarily associate with the realms of conjugal reproduction: the market (consumerism) and the state ('big brother'). In fact, much of the Euro-American history of kinship has been concerned with tracing the development of a *separation* between this private domain and the public domains of the market and state (Strathern 1992a: 103–4, 187–92). This suggests that the conception of limits intrinsic to Euro-American kinship is not in fact as separate from these other domains as first appears.

Kinship implies a form of regulation. What is implicitly being regulated according to informants' images are the 'biological foundations' of the relationships referred to here as 'family' and 'relatives'. This was the image that Winnie and Ted Murphy were struggling with in articulating their respective roles as step-parent (no biological connection) and parent (biological tie). When the foundations are imagined as no longer regulated, concern is expressed: for example, the possibility that techniques of anonymous donation could conceivably enable a brother's sperm to be received by his sister. This particular potentiality became visible to Winnie and Ted at the end of our discussion. I had referred to concerns people had expressed in Alltown:

WM: They couldn't possibly make that kind of error surely, like my brother could go along and donate sperm and I could innocently pick that sperm up? There must be some kind of regulation.

And Ted immediately follows:

TM: The only way you could do that is knowing the name of the donor isn't it? I had never thought of that you know. This thing about incest really throws all the thing out, all the things we've been saying about, Oh yes, we'd come to terms with that, then you throw it in, you don't know who the donors are. We've been saying we shouldn't know who the donor is because it makes life easier for everybody else.

In the everyday thoughts and perceptions of the couples reported here (as more generally), family and kinship is conceived as a domain separate from wider political and economic structures. However, when assumptions underlying conceptions of family and kinship are made explicit, their intrinsic connection with the domains of market and state becomes visible. In other words, when the basis of our most familiar relationships come to appear potentially unregulated, then political and economic domains, by virtue of this intrinsic connection, become so as well.

Debates about the regulation of the market, as much as those about regulating the state, are public and wide-ranging. We do not think twice about offering an opinion as to whether more regulation or less is desirable. What is less evident, even hidden, is the manner in which these debates imply a particular conception of relatedness that we commonly understand as family and kinship. In this way, the concern of Denis White expressed in the previous section, and of other informants, is a genuine concern. As debated by the parliamentarians reported in the next chapter, or as discerned by clinicians (Chapter 1), medical developments are racing ahead of the ordinary man and woman. As Denis sees this, it takes time to catch up with these changes and in the process our thoughts are transformed. Yet perhaps it is not just our thoughts that are changing, in the way Denis suggests, but the previously *implicit* contexts to which they have to be *explicitly* focused, and the images by which they are summoned.

We have seen, through the material presented in this chapter, that men and women struggle to sustain a perspective on the present in the face of innovations that seem to threaten their accepted ideas and practices. In the future, NRT might be more readily available and 'acceptable', but it will not be 'our' thinking and practices that have necessarily changed as a result so much as the areas and domains where they are *visibly* applied. These are issues that will continue to be debated, both politically and ethically – framed by the agencies of the market and state – and to which concepts of family and kinship will remain intrinsically connected.

NOTES

1 I was reminded of this passage in Harvey (1989) by a productive comment from Ronnie Frankenberg at the September 1991 workshop.
2 It should be noted here that it would be mistaken to conclude from the material presented below that informants were opposed completely (with exceptions noted) to the development of NRT, or to its take-up by the general public. What are being highlighted are connections made explicit by NRT, to domains conventionally conceived as separate from kinship and family. The concerns expressed are as much a product of the connections being made visible as they are of the connections themselves.
3 Here, Strathern is referring to what she calls the second 'fact' of modern kinship; the first 'fact' is the individuality of persons (1992a: 14), while the third 'fact' is that individuals reproduce individuals (1992a: 53).
4 The families for the ESRC-PICT research project were initially recruited

through local schools. Contact was made through the head teacher who was asked to recommend families for participation in the research. An initial meeting was then arranged, at which time the families could decide whether they wanted to participate further in the research.

5 Allen Abramson (personal communication) has suggested that one of the recurring themes *implicitly* at work in this sub-text is the 'self-externalization of parental biology in one's own children'. I would argue that this conceptualisation becomes *explicit* in the light of NRT. As a number of informants indicated, it is taken for granted until one is 'confronted with the possibility it could not be your child' (see p. 107, above; cf. Schneider (1992) for an insightful discussion and elaboration of these processes). I am grateful to Allen Abramson for his very helpful comments on this chapter.

6 Jeanette Edwards, personal communication. I am grateful to her for comments on this chapter.

7 Had this study been intended as a contribution to the sociology of the family, then it would have been appropriate to elicit material from the perspective of other families, or to have contextualised the present selection in relation to them.

8 Several men and women evoked the example of Louise Brown in the discussions (see below). It is significant to note that she has become a cultural icon for what is possible for *people*: her introduction into a number of discussions is first and foremost because she can be cited as a real human being.

9 Both Rajni and Ganesh could imagine, under strict moral constraints, the increased take-up of NRT in British society. However, Ganesh insisted that, in Indian culture, the possibility of anonymous genetic material would not be thinkable: 'Now they want to know, if it's an anonymous sperm, will you know which caste it comes from? So it's completely out of the question, they will never accept it. Never accept it, even if they are given 100 per cent verity it's a high caste, they still won't accept it.'

10 I mention this here to caution against a reading of the narratives presented here as corresponding to the views associated with either 'men' or 'women'.

11 Ted's conception of surrogacy in this instance was based on the use of the surrogate's eggs as well as her womb.

12 I have indicated the religious affiliations for several of the couples reported here. Only in the case of the De Guys, however, did religious beliefs become an explicit and inhibiting issue with respect to the topics of this research.

13 Except in the one family where religious principle prevailed.

ACKNOWLEDGEMENT

I would like to thank the women and men who allowed me into their homes to discuss the topics reported in this chapter. All their names have been changed.

Afterword for Chapter 3

Glimpses of moments in the 'circuit of culture'

Eric Hirsch

In reflecting on this chapter my attention was drawn towards notions of regulation. The reasons for this focus, as I intend to indicate briefly, illustrate some of the wider implications of this chapter as well as the volume as a whole.

The research for the present chapter was conducted shortly after I had completed a study focused on the domestic environment of information and communication technologies (ICT) (see Hirsch 1992, 1998c cf. Hirsch 1998a).[1] That first study was conducted at a time when a new regulatory environment was being implemented for the provision of television, cable, telecommunication and other ICT (see Baldwin *et al.* 1996).

'De-regulation', as it was (and still is) called (Thompson 1997), meant that previously separate technological systems and their distinct forms of regulation – as with television broadcasting, or telecommunications – would now be opened to greater competition. Part of the rationale for this change was that it would enable greater individual 'choice' and the potential for technological convergence (see Hirsch 1998b). Concern was expressed at the time, as it still is today, that such changes would lead to the alteration of our traditional forms of domestic culture, regulated so as to conform to national standards of taste and public service. Instead, standardised, market-led products would become the staple diet of ICT users, conforming to the global corporate plans of a Murdoch or Disney.

This tension between the established, traditional and regulated, in contrast to new forms of potentially unregulated change, emerged as a central theme in the discussions reported here, concerned as they are with the new reproductive technologies (NRT). What is of particular interest is that the potential lack of regulation, suggested by the innovations made possible by NRT, evoked idioms of rampant consumerism and extreme forms of control and power; idioms also recurrently evoked in the debates surrounding the de-regulated environment of ICT (Thompson 1997: 14).

We have here, then, concerns about regulation[2] in what are conventionally perceived as separate domains of culture (i.e. ICT and NRT). Although perceived as separate domains they also have the capacity to appear connected (through the evocation of an analogous set of idioms) when the (regulatory) conventions which keep them separate seem to be removed. Similarly, English culture is envisaged as separated into distinct domains, but is simultaneously all of a piece.

One of the concluding themes of this chapter is that domains such as the market or state are perceived as separate, and only appear as connected when our taken-for-granted relationships seem to have lost their regulated basis. Notions of relatedness (kinship) are thus pervasive but can remain circumscribed or hidden with respect to other domains of culture. As Strathern notes here (p. 198), Euro-American kinship contains both relational and non-relational ways of thinking about persons. Kinship can thus 'appear' and 'disappear'; persons can appear as autonomous, separate entities, or as entities enmeshed in social relationships.

This conclusion is of particular interest when considered in relation to a recent set of texts (in a series entitled 'Culture, Media and Identities'[3] – hereafter CMI), which have as their central model what is referred to as the 'circuit of culture'. This is depicted as a set of separate but interrelated 'moments' comprising representation, identity, production, consumption and regulation. Each volume focuses on a specific moment of this circuit, at once highlighting the separateness of the moment and its simultaneous connection with all the other moments. The Sony Walkman is used as an exemplary cultural artefact to illustrate this circuit, as documented in the first volume. What I find of interest about this project is the manner in which the authors can describe the moments as once separate and interconnected (visualised in graphic form; Thompson 1997: 3). The problem addressed by this project is not to consider how such a cultural process ('circuit') is conceivable and readily comprehended, but to show how it operates:

> It has been suggested that in order to gain a *full understanding* of any cultural text or artefact, such as the Sony Walkman, it is necessary to analyze the processes of representation, identity, production, consumption and regulation. A cultural artefact like the Walkman has an impact upon the regulation of social life through the ways in which it is represented, the identities associated with it, and the articulation of its production and consumption.
>
> (Thompson 1997: 2; emphasis added)

Thus if we focus on regulation, for example, issues such as the transgression of public and private boundaries come into view as persons privately listen to music in public contexts where this was previously not practised. When the Walkman first appeared, issues about its proper regulation were much publicised, but its use now appears part of accepted everyday, even 'traditional', routines.

What if we were to suggest that there were two equally important dimensions linked to the proper understanding of the 'circuit of culture's' operation. One concerns our capacity to switch from the moments of the circuit of culture as at once separate and as inter-connected. And the second concerns our capacity to see this in an almost self-evident manner.

What are these various moments of the circuit of culture? They are particular contexts of personal and/or collective agency and action – where persons are both relational and non-relational. If we focus, for example, on regulation in the case of NRT we bring into focus the complex series of debates reported in Mulkay's (1997) book. Mulkay documents how various modes of representation were deployed by the pro- and anti- lobbies, how particular versions were produced in the media for popular consumption and how these positions resonated with the identities of the persons involved, or the public more generally. In fact Mulkay frames his portrayal of the 'embryo research debate' in terms of 'cultural tensions' (1997: 3, 131) and a motivating sense of 'cultural nostalgia' (1997: 170). We could, it seems, even speak of the 'culture of NRT', its specific 'circuit', and our capacity to switch between its various moments.

Stuart Hall, in his concluding chapter to the CMI project, argues that culture has now become central both at a local level and on a global scale. Whereas previously we might have asked whether culture and its transformations were determined by the economy, market, state and so on, we now see matters in terms of mutual determinations:

> what is being argued . . . is not that 'everything is culture' but that every social practice depends on or relates to meaning; consequently, that culture is one of the constitutive conditions of existence of that practice, that every social practice has a cultural dimension.
>
> (Hall 1997: 225–6; cf. Strathern 1995: 161)

Just as culture has become more visible, so have issues concerning its regulation and who is seen to govern its regulation, particularly when de-regulation and choice are so much to the fore. Hall speaks of the inter-related nature of the regulation *of* culture and regulation *by* culture. An increasing set of diverse contexts like ICT and NRT are perceived as 'cultural' and subject, as they are, to explicit forms of regulation (or de-regulation, as the case may be). In addition, persons are now being asked to exercise more self-regulation as with the enterprising individual and their greater individual choice (Hall 1997: 233–236).

How, it may be asked, have we been enabled to perceive these transformations – to visualise them? Has there been a shift from the person seen as enmeshed in an overarching form of societal regulation to one where the ground has shifted to focus on the individual, i.e. from cultural regulation to self-regulation? What the CMI project appears to lack is a sustained examination of the Euro-American person and the relationality of such personhood, which anthropologists refer to as kinship. Reading the discussions of the couples described in this chapter we catch glimpses of all the 'moments' in the 'circuit of culture', each from the different vantage points of their respective domestic contexts. We can at once see the moments as separate, then seemingly connected. What has enabled this perceptual switching? I would suggest it is the person's capacity both to conceive and to imagine a world of separate individuals/entities and of interrelated individuals/entities. The men and women speak here, at one instance, of a world of unregulated relationships. At another instance, though, the conventions of regulated relationships – analogous to a regulated culture – appear firmly in place.

The present chapter, then, read in conjunction with its partner chapters, is a powerful example of Marcus's (1995) call for 'multi-sited ethnography'. This innovative feature of the book can only be read together with the English description of persons and relations contained by the book. It is *their* 'multi-sitedness' – at once appearing enmeshed in networks of relations, multiple roles and overlapping contexts, and then appearing as an autonomous entity, occupying a singular role and detached from other sites and contexts.

In this regard the call for multi-sited ethnography is of a piece with the 'circuit of culture' project. To suggest this is not to deny their relevance to contemporary concerns or provocations to research. Rather, it is to argue that the relevance of the present chapter, as with the book as a whole, should not be confined within debates about NRT and its socio-cultural implications. This is particularly the case when kinship can at once appear of the utmost significance and then seem to disappear without trace. The analysis reported here provides an important perspective on English personhood and relations – kinship – and suggests that kinship and its transformations need to be at the centre of debates concerning social and cultural theory and the centre of methods and practice of socio-cultural research.

NOTES

1 Sixteen families participated in the earlier study; twelve of those same families are reported here.
2 Regulation here entails both the conduct of commercial and non-commercial relations; the distinction between them is increasingly blurred with respect both to NRT and ICT.
3 The series contains the following volumes, all published by Sage during 1997: *Doing Cultural Studies: The Story of the Sony Walkman*, P. du Gay, S. Hall, L. Janes, H. Mackay and K. Negus; *Representation: Cultural Representations and Signifying Practices*, S. Hall (ed.); *Identity and Difference*, K. Woodward (ed.); *Production of Culture/Cultures of Production*, P. du Gay (ed.); *Consumption and Everyday life*, H. Mackay (ed.); *Media and Cultural Regulation*, K. Thompson (ed.).

4 Making representations

The parliamentary debate on the Human Fertilisation and Embryology Act

Sarah Franklin

This chapter presents findings from analysis of a particular set of representations of kinship in the context of new reproductive technologies (NRTs). These are the parliamentary debates accompanying the passage into law of the British government's Human Fertilisation and Embryology Bill, introduced in November 1989 and enacted in November 1990. Following a brief contextualisation of these debates and a discussion of the analytic procedures undertaken, I present an analysis of the official records from *Hansard*. The findings are organised with respect to three analytical perspectives: (1) the ways in which the debates can be read from an anthropological perspective as a formal, public negotiation of kinship; (2) the implications of such a perspective for an understanding of the framing and grounding of the terms of public debate, and thus future debates; and (3) the implications for anthropological understandings of kinship which may be seen to derive from the particular representations of kinship produced in these debates.

This exercise is therefore a reflexive one; it presumes a two-way traffic. Analytic perspectives unfamiliar to the mode of debate are introduced, as are elements of the debate unfamiliar to the mode of analysis. The object of enquiry is thus itself relational, dually constituted by contrasting modes of 'making sense'.

THE CONTEXT: A CONCEPTUAL VACUUM

As we saw in Chapter 1, the origin of the legislative process which led to the enactment of the Human Fertilisation and Embryology Bill (now Act, hereafter referred to as the HFEB) is frequently attributed to a birth: 'the birth of Louise Brown'. This world-famous birth in Oldham, Lancashire, was not in itself remarkable. Rather, its significance lay in its confirmation of the viability of a mode of conception which had occurred nine months earlier: in vitro fertilisation (IVF); she was a 'test tube baby'. Her birth thus signalled the advent of radical and unprecedented conceptive possibilities. The scope of these possibilities continues to expand. In addition to new conceptive techniques, the removal of eggs from a woman's body (the most difficult initial obstacle to successful IVF) has facilitated many other interventions into the process of procreation. The medical and clinical context of these developments is outlined in Chapter 1. Alongside the technology came new opportunities to investigate, by means of direct observation and research previously unavailable to natural scientists and clinicians, the process of early embryonic development. In turn, these opportunities were seen to offer much therapeutic and experimental potential, and to open up whole new vistas of knowledge. Through IVF, a form of infertility treatment unique (and so named) for its creation of an embryo outside the body, a new 'era' of reproduction was seen to emerge. It is this 'reproductive revolution' which was seen to originate in the birth of Louise Brown.

Following this novel parturition, the British government began a series of proceedings aimed to establish clear regulatory guidelines controlling embryo research and thereby aspects of infertility services. Several potentialities were seen to be at stake: new research and technology; new persons and new beings in the form of embryos; new facts and new knowledges; and new risks of possible misuses of the techniques. Reproductive futures in this context emerged as a set of complex and unfamiliar issues. This legislative trajectory drew on existing law to some extent, but in large part comprised an unprecedented legislative initiative to govern 'human fertilisation and embryology'. The birth of Louise Brown bought into being more than a child; it created a 'legislative vacuum' that needed to be filled.

The perspective of legislation

The legislative process can be understood to be composed of three main parts: consultation with the general public and diverse recognised bodies of opinion and advice (e.g. expert, professional, religious, voluntary and charitable); the drafting of proposed legislation by government officials; and parliamentary debate on Bills and Reports. Different kinds of information, facts, knowledge, opinion and expertise were thus brought together, in accordance with established procedures and conventions, in the attempt to formulate a consensual basis for regulation of new forms of assisted reproduction. The general public, the government and Parliament each had a role in the enactment of legislation which was, optimally, intended to represent to the most democratic degree possible the outcome of the input of all three.

The first landmark in the effort to redress the 'legislative vacuum' brought into existence by the birth of Louise Brown was the commissioning in 1982 of the Committee of Inquiry into Human Fertilisation and Embryology by Norman Tebbit, then a Minister. The Committee, headed by Mary Warnock and subsequently known as the Warnock Committee, published its Report in 1984. The recommendations of its Report are divided into 5 sections: A, the licensing body and its functions; B, principles of provision; C, service provision; D, legal limits on research; and E, legal changes. In sum, the Warnock Committee's recommendations covered three areas: infertility services; the status of children born of new techniques; and embryo research. These recommendations were debated in the House of Lords in 1984, thus initiating the parliamentary proceedings which are the subject of this analysis. Close on the heels of the parliamentary debate of the Warnock Report came the Surrogacy Arrangements Act, banning commercial surrogacy, and a Private Member's Bill from MP Enoch Powell, entitled the Unborn Children (Protection) Bill. This Bill was debated in the 1985–86 parliamentary session and, though defeated, led to the establishment of a powerful medical/scientific lobby which opposed a ban on embryo research. The government also produced a Consultation Paper in 1986, aimed to elicit reactions from the general public and appropriate public bodies. In 1987, the government published a White Paper outlining proposed legislation. This eventually became the Human Fertilisation and Embryology Bill which was introduced into Parliament in the autumn of 1989.[1]

Importantly, then, one of the first major parliamentary debates subsequent to the Warnock Report concerned embryo research. The somewhat unexpected (for example, by Warnock) prominence of 'the embryo question' also prompted the government to undertake a drafting innovation specific to this issue, a so-called 'conscience vote' on embryo research (Clause 11). Members of Parliament were offered a choice between two clauses, one banning embryo research and one permitting it subject to strict regulations.[2]

The HFEB began its parliamentary passage, then, twelve years after the event from which it was said to have originated. This long delay is but one of many indicators of the unique challenges such legislation presented to the various interested parties involved. Following its introduction into Parliament in November 1989, the Bill went through several stages, which are outlined here for reference purposes. The first major debate on the Bill was the Second Reading in the House of Lords on 7 December 1989, during which speakers addressed themselves to the Bill as a whole.[3] It went into Committee in the House of Lords in February of 1990 where specific clause amendments were debated. The Committee stage was followed by the Report stage in which further amendments were debated, in March 1990, after which it was given its Third Reading in the House of Lords before being passed and sent to the House of Commons. Following the opening debate of the Bill in the House of Commons on 2 April 1990, it went through two committee stages. The first, a Committee of the Whole House, consisted of debate on two issues only, those of embryo research and abortion (23 and 24 April). Subsequently, in May 1990, the Bill went into a Standing Committee for debate on the rest of the clauses. In June, two days were devoted to the report from the Standing Committee, after which the Bill was returned to the House of Lords, amended and agreed to, on 22 June 1990. Further amendments were decided upon in the House of Lords in October 1990, shortly before the Bill received Royal Assent and was thus enacted on 1 November 1990.

It is the *Official Record* of these debates which constitutes my data set. The data thus consist of a lengthy text: a transcript of formal, public debate of human fertilisation and embryology as reported in the House of Lords' and the House of Commons' *Hansard*. Most narrowly, this text is a record of formal parliamentary debate. To the anthropologist, however, the parliamentary debate involved in the passage of the HFEB provides a window on the contemporary negotiation of kinship ties and obligations. From this perspective, the parliamentary debate was a unique instance of formal, public kinship negotiation. In this context, kinship meanings normally operative at the level of assumed common sense, or taken-for-granted obviousness, were by necessity made explicit. Moreover, the perceived threat to existing kinship foundations, such as the ideal of the 'traditional' (nuclear, biological) family, precipitated animated discussion of the importance of this ideal, its key ingredients, boundaries, and so forth. To the anthropologist familiar with kinship theory, the parliamentary debate of the HFEA could be seen as sharing much in common with debates in other cultures, in previous historical periods in this culture,[4] and indeed within the discipline of anthropology itself.

The perspective of anthropology

Given the longstanding importance to anthropology of the cultural construction or negotiation of conception and parenthood, it is somewhat surprising that more anthropological interest has not been focused on recent public debate such as that conducted in Parliament. This neglect is undoubtedly related to the underdevelopment of anthropological study concerning kinship in contemporary Euro-American culture more generally.[5] To date, anthropological study of public debate concerning kinship in the context of NRTs is minimal.

An important exception at the outset of parliamentary proceedings was Rivière's (1985) contribution. His article, entitled 'Unscrambling parenthood', reflected on the reproductive dilemmas encountered in the Warnock Report and the Powell Bill. Rivière's central argument, that these would be familiar to anthropologists, emphasised a history of kinship theory in which a distinction between social and natural parenthood had long been utilised.

Rivière's claim, that the dilemmas encountered in public and parliamentary debates of NRTs would be familiar to anthropologists, has also proved true of the later debates, and can be productively extended to encompass several of their dimensions. Many of the classic elements of kinship study may be recognised in these debates, including: beliefs about conception and personhood; prescriptions concerning marriage, inheritance and descent; the symbolic significance of shared bodily substance; and the social construction of natural facts. By examining the parliamentary negotiations from these established perspectives of kinship analysis, it becomes clear not only why they are of interest to anthropologists, but also why anthropological perspectives might be of consequence to the terms of debate. Given the widely acknowledged difficulties surrounding the question of how the terms of debate were/are to be established, the uncertainty surrounding their formulation, and the inevitability of many, likely to be even more challenging, future debates, anthropologists and parliamentarians can indeed be seen to have something in common in the effort to elucidate the foundations of kinship.[6]

A more recent and substantial anthropological study in Britain concerning these areas is that of Cannell (1990), who examines the contested notion of 'the family' in the context of public debate over both the Warnock Report and the 1985 campaign by Victoria Gillick in the English courts to prevent doctors from prescribing contraceptives to girls under 16 years of age without their parents' consent. Examining the complex interplay of media imagery in these debates, Cannell contrasts the spectre of reproduction without sex via NRTs, with the possibility of sex without reproduction enabled by contraceptive technology. In both debates, she concludes, it is the 'single ideological terrain' of the 'naturalness of the family' which is presupposed as under threat. Hence, both debates, though productive of moral panic, and of contradictory enunciations of 'traditional family values', were, Cannell argues, occasions though which a shared discourse affirming these values, and grounding them in 'nature' were restored.

It should be noted at the outset, then, that both the analytic procedures and the data set utilised in this chapter constitute an intervention into an area as yet hardly approached by anthropologists.[7]

It is in part a consequence of this novelty that the chapter initially divides into sections. The first section, 'Familiar kinship', develops upon Rivière's analysis to elaborate those aspects of the parliamentary debate most familiar to anthropologists from the perspective of established kinship theory and the ethnographic record. In the subsequent section, 'Unfamiliar kinship', some implications of the debate for anthropological understandings of kinship are suggested. In the conclusion, these are brought together in a discussion of the relevance of anthropology for future public debates concerning kinship in the context of the NRTs.

FAMILIAR KINSHIP

The significance of assumptions about conception to the cultural construction of kinship and personhood is well established within anthropological concerns. In historic debates in anthropology, such as the 'virgin birth' controversy,[8] conception accounts are seen to provide an important source of evidence about the foundations of not only kinship but the social order and cosmology. The respective contributions of other persons to one's own personal origins provide the foundations for social ties and obligations, and make evident foundational premises about the world. As definitions of what makes a person, they reveal (to the outsider) important cultural anchors and prescriptions for relationships in general, as well as those immediately brought into being at birth.

Both Rivière's and Cannell's arguments build on such established anthropological conventions of understanding kinship in order to elucidate the source of moral panic surrounding technological intervention into the reproductive process. In their respective analyses, both confirm the importance of kinship constructs at a symbolic level, and explicate the degree of public concern aroused by the spectre of reproductive intervention accordingly. Yet re-inscribing current public debate over reproductive intervention on the template of established anthropological certainties concerning kinship is variably enabling. In Rivière's case, it allows the debate over Warnock to be put into a wider perspective, with the aim of alleviating panic. The implication is that 'we' (the British) are engaged in something familiar, universal and even traditional: the negotiation of the social and natural facts of kinship. In Cannell's case, too, the analysis confirms the purchase of anthropological assessments: 'we' (the anthropologists) have a discursive technology to describe what is occurring – it is called 'kinship'.

This dual tendency to reassure by confirming both the basic human importance of kinship debates and the capacity of anthropology to translate moral panic into an ordered proceeding, through naming it and defining it according to conventional disciplinary wisdom, was entirely befitting to the occasion of such debates. So explicit were these recent public debates in their foregrounding of the condensed nodes of meaning familiar to anthropologists, so classic was the character of their components, such an analytic tendency was, indeed, almost irresistible. The opportunity of matching certain features of current public debate with the explanatory mode provided by anthropology informed much of the early period of my own analysis as described in this chapter. In the end, however, it proved insufficient. I first briefly outline some of the most important characteristics of public debate which initially confirmed such an approach.

Conception and personhood

One notable feature of the parliamentary debates from this perspective is their saturation with conception litanies. These formulaic accounts of the sequence of events involved in embryogenesis punctuate the debates with a frequency and urgency that bring to mind familiar examples from the ethnographic record, such as Malinowski's classic accounts (1927, 1930) from the Trobriand Islands. Though exclusively dedicated to the narrow legal question of the status of the embryo for the purposes of state regulation affecting it, these conception litanies, with their explicit concern for the personhood of the embryo, clearly represented much wider concerns, indeed no less than the definitions of morality, humanity and society.

Despite their fundamental opposition, advocates of both positions in 'the embryo debate' had much in common in perceiving it as the nodal point of wider contestations. As in the case of people in Alltown, opposing views arose from different perspectives on values held in common (Chapter 2). Parliamentarians shared certain assumptions concerning which facts about the embryo were to be considered most important. Most significant among the shared definitions of embryonic 'personhood' were its biogenetic basis and the unique individuality of which this was seen to be definitive. Anti-embryo-research parliamentarians argued that fertilisation is the moment when personhood is established because of the presence of its 'unique genetic blueprint', formed by the union of the chromosomal material of the two gametes, egg and sperm, which denoted the presence of a new individual human being. Pro-embryo-research parliamentarians argued that until the formation of the 'primitive streak' (the emergent spinal column), visible at approximately fourteen days, the embryo was not a distinct individual. Even those who argued a religious (notably Catholic) position that 'life begins at conception' did so on the basis that the formation of 'a unique genetic blueprint' was evidence of the equivalent of ensoulment, a position which could be described as a biotheological one (see Ford 1988). In agreement about the ingredients of personhood – an identifiable 'starting point' defined as the emergence of a distinct individual biogenetic potential for development – the two sides disagreed over the exact point at which this occurred.

Such a concept of personhood has direct implications for many areas of debate other than embryo research. In establishing biogenetic individuality as the basis of personhood, it contributes to what can be described as the geneticisation of both kinship and identity. Children born of donation were debated in terms of their right to know their genetic origins, a right seen as integral to their successful development and acquisition of a complete identity. A concept such as 'genetic identity' would confirm an anthropological reading of the specific importance of biogenetic facts in Euro-American culture: a child's conception has a powerful symbolic importance to cultural constructions of kinship and personhood. This reading would also partly explain the deep reluctance of many parliamentarians to abandon the principle of maintaining the genetic accuracy of the Birth Registry.

The ability to define personhood in strictly biogenetic terms is consistent with the primary kinship unit of the biological family, the primary kinship distinction between 'blood' relations and in-laws, the bilateral reckoning of relations, and the rules concerning incest in contemporary English kinship. Such readings of the parliamentary debate would be familiar indeed to the anthropologist, who might easily confirm the importance of beliefs about conception to the construction of kinship.

The social construction of natural facts

The parliamentary debates surrounding the HFEB were also significant in terms of anthropological understandings of the symbolic functions of the so-called biological facts of sexual reproduction. This has proved an increasingly important trajectory within recent kinship theory, particularly where it has intersected with feminist anthropological understandings of gender (see Collier and Yanagisako 1987). This trajectory has its roots in the anthropological model that takes the biological fact of genetic inheritance as a culturally specific explanation of relatedness. Such an explanation is irrelevant, inadequate, or merely partial in many other constructions of kinship ties with different cultural origins. That the biological facts hold such a prominent position in Euro-American kinship definitions therefore requires more explanation than that they are 'true' (see Schneider 1968). It requires that they be located in the context of a conceptual system organised to confirm their cultural legitimacy and explanatory purchase.

The parliamentary debates suggest that this exercise may be more challenging than we initially assumed, due to the blurring of boundaries around the difference between a 'natural fact' and assisted nature in the context of assisted reproduction. In any event, were one engaged in the attempt to elucidate the character of kinship in contemporary Euro-American cultures, the significance of 'the biological facts of sexual reproduction' could not be underestimated. A single example here will suffice.

As we have seen, the debate over embryo research resulted from a division of strongly felt opinion less in terms of *how* the embryo might be regarded as a person, than *when* it became so. Contested on the terrain of state-of-the-art embryology, debate came to focus particularly upon one key 'natural fact' of embryogenesis, namely, the formation of the so-called 'primitive streak'. Here was a marker, a natural dividing point, which would serve as a basis for a legislative distinction between permissible and impermissible research.

A 'boundary' found in 'nature' and duly classified by biological science (in the form of the distinction between the embryo and the 'pre-embryo' – a much contested term) conforms fully to the structural requirements of Euro-American kinship systems, at least if we take as an example that elucidated by Schneider for American culture (1968). That is, the order of nature provides the basis or foundation for the order of law in the definition of kinship ties. True to the consistent attribution of privileged authority to clinical and scientific expertise throughout the debates, 'natural facts' such as the primitive streak were seen to provide the neutral, impartial and objective facts of the matter upon which legislation should properly be based.[9]

While this kind of framework for negotiating kinship meanings is familiar to anthropological debate, there arise some interesting discrepancies in relation to the law itself. Here, the primitive streak is 'to be taken to have appeared in an embryo not later than the end of the period of fourteen days' (HFEB, Section 3). In other words, although it provides the natural justification for a legal limit on research, the *actual* appearance of the primitive streak is legally irrelevant, having been displaced by a more clearly defined unit of measurement: 'the period of fourteen days'. Hence, the authority of natural facts becomes indeterminate. The law is, in fact, indifferent to their permutations. Insufficient as a foundation for legal certainty or authority, the biological facts are displaced.

Such a displacement, though perhaps seemingly minor in itself, invokes a tension at the heart of the attempt to legislate in an area defined as 'natural', and seen to be founded upon the authority of biological science. The problem is that nature is assisted. It was this 'assistance' (to conception) which brought a legislative vacuum into being. Having 'failed', 'nature' (in the form of Louise Brown's mother's 'failed' reproductive organs) was 'given a helping hand' by Robert Edwards and Patrick Steptoe, thus producing an assisted conception. Nature thus becomes *a mediated authority*, a partial foundation, and then in need of further 'assistance' by the law to confirm its certainty. Nature is thus doubly mediated: it is interpreted by its assistants, the scientists and clinicians whose expert advice was the basis for parliamentary decision-making, and it is then rendered arbitrary by the law once its 'design' has been revealed. Thus the law makes residual what it claims as its foundation: it renders uncertain the very premise of its certainty.

Two counterposed processes can be seen to be at work: the displacement of 'natural facts' by social decision-making (the period of fourteen days), and the displacement of social facts by biology. In some cases, the authority of nature has been completely lost, as in elucidation of 'the meaning of mother':

> The woman who is carrying or has carried a child as a result of the placing in her of an embryo or of sperm and eggs, and no other woman, is to be treated as the mother of the child.
>
> (HFEB, S.27)

Here, the dilemma of assisted nature resides in the emergence of two 'natural' mothers: the genetic mother and the birth mother. Who is the 'real' mother? Nature cannot referee. In other cases, the authority of nature was simply abandoned, as in the case of gamete donors whose 'natural' parenthood was rendered legally unrecognisable. Likewise, in the granting to husbands of women recipients of DI the right to register their name as father on the birth certificate, the law takes on new powers of conferring parental status (see HFEB, Section 28).

To argue simply that the law in such cases explicitly supersedes (or 'assists') in the social construction of natural facts to an unprecedented degree is not enough, since, by definition, a law designed to establish regulatory control over 'human fertilisation and embryology' could do little else. To recognise that there is a fundamental tension between the social construction of the domain of the natural as an independent force and authority unto itself, and its (dual) assistance to make it explicitly so is merely to confirm an already established – though in this instance delightfully baroque – habit of cultural practice. One might also consider the pronounced degree to which the debate over matters which would be readily identifiable to an anthropologist as relational, such as the acquisition of identity or the definition of parenthood, are debated in Parliament in the asocial, non-relational discourse of biological facts. Finally, there is a certain paradoxical dimension to the debates, in that this displacement of kinship or sociality among persons is undertaken alongside the granting of all sorts of personal, social and relational attributes to eggs, sperm, zygotes, concepti and other micro-entities.

On the face of it, such observations seem amenable to analysis based on established anthropological understandings of kinship. Indeed, much that is interesting and useful can be said about what is immediately recognisable as representations of 'kinship' in the context of NRTs in the parliamentary debates. Also on the face of it, it might seem rather doubtful how much one could communicate about the relevance of such observations to a parliamentarian or a (non-anthropological) 'layperson'. None the less, a case could be made for the value of such expertise to public debate. The familiarity of anthropologists with the precise matters of kinship adjudication at stake would appear to confirm the existing expertise of the discipline, simply by demonstrating how anthropology 'makes sense' of these debates in terms of its specialist conventions of explication. But the matter does not rest there.

UNFAMILIAR KINSHIP

> The embryo at conception is indeed a marvellous minute cell and those like me who have seen it for the first time have been struck by a sense of awe. As Professor Edwards remarked when he looked at Louise Brown at the four cell stage: 'It looked beautiful.'
>
> (The Duke of Norfolk, HL, 7.12.89, c. 1031)

> It is a little late to be saying that man should not interfere with nature or try to help it on a little. . . . In any case, the problem is different now; nature needs our help if it is to survive what has already been done to it.
>
> (Lord Flowers, HL, 7.12.89, c. 1061)

While it is possible to consider the parliamentary debates in terms of established anthropological approaches to kinship, such as those outlined in the previous section, this possibility also presents a dilemma. There is a gap between those aspects of debate which are most recognisably about kinship to the anthropologist, and those aspects of debate most significant to parliamentarians. What is (or is not) recognised as kinship in the context of public and parliamentary debates over NRTs must be translated into what is anthropologically recognisable as kinship, and then translated back again. Anthropology offers one mode of understanding: 'they are really talking about kinship'. By so doing, however, it renders kinship only eruditely recognisable. It therefore creates a problem for itself in seeking common ground upon which kinship might be more mutually visible.

There is a parallel dilemma: an exemplary one. What is most recognisable as kinship to parliamentarians (where they speak explicitly of 'kinship') is in the least significant parts of the debate, concerning inheritances of clan chieftainships and other similarly esoteric matters. What is most important to parliamentarians in the debate is least recognisable as kinship to anthropologists; that is, the embryo debates, in which the individuated, non-relational pre-person prevails. The gap between the anthropologists' and the parliamentarians' interest in recognising kinship would appear to grow in proportion to the centrality (to the legislation) of the subject under debate.

In sum, one is repeatedly struck by the non-relational character of parliamentary debate. It might even be considered some kind of unique cultural achievement to have spent so much time talking about such obviously relational matters – parenthood, marriage, the family, the desire for children – in a manner which makes kinship and relationships invisible. In fact, as if this were even deliberate, the only place where concrete relationships *are* discussed, those between donor children and their genetic parents, the aim is to ensure (by preserving anonymity) that a relationship never exists. Moreover, one of the main problems encountered in the search for 'representations of kinship' in the parliamentary debates surrounding the HFEB is that the debate is not only suffused in the non-relational language of biology, but is mostly concerned with the rights and status of embryos, whose primary potential is to (a) become independently viable, and (b) become an individual.

These are not the only grounds for a shift in focus. If an understanding of the character of kinship represented in the parliamentary debates would seem to require partial redefinition, or re-recognition, of 'what kinship is all about', the impetus to do so can also be drawn from within anthropology itself, where solid kinship has melted into thin air on more than one occasion.

Familiar kinship revisited

One might provide a brief account of its history by describing the relational character of the concept of kinship itself, for it has always served as a productively contestable episteme in anthropology. The discipline has been argued to have kinship at its 'core', the classification of lineage systems having been original to the study of other cultures, and to what is now known as modern(ist) anthropology. In relation to the 'savage' peoples of nineteenth-century anthropologising, classificatory kinship was initially seen as a measure of degrees of evolution towards civilisation. For the most assiduous early-twentieth-century critic of this early model, Malinowski, kinship in its social and biological varieties was the universal institution linking all mankind. To the later structural-functionalists, kinship became the definitive instrument of social order in traditional cultures, mediating between the domestic and jural domains, and providing the functions served by the workplace and the state in 'modern' societies. With the decline of the structural-functionalist model in the 1960s, kinship studies also diminished in significance within anthropology.

If few kinship studies have been undertaken of contemporary Euro-American cultures, the most significant resurgence of kinship theory derives from one of them, Schneider's account of American kinship. Here, kinship shifts into the realm of the symbolic, resurfacing with the rise of cultural anthropology once again transformed. Hence it acquires renewed currency, most recently in speculative offerings to effect a merger between kinship and gender studies (Collier and Yanagisako 1987).

It is the basis of the latter union which suggests a possible shift in focus whereby kinship could be refigured in order to ground a different approach to 'the representation of kinship in the context of the new reproductive technology' in the parliamentary debates. Collier and Yanagisako (1987) argue that the problem with kinship studies, even in their Schneiderian vein, is that they take for granted what most needs explaining, which are the 'facts' of sexual reproduction. In other words, the primary fact of sexual difference itself is not self-evident. Hence the turn to theories of gender, where this question also holds a privileged place.

Taken in a different direction, one might view the parliamentary debates from this starting point. What if the question were not that of finding a mutually recognisable kinship, but a mutually *unrecognisable* one? By forfeiting existing anthropological understandings of kinship, and recognising that we are looking at 'unfamiliar kinship', there is at least the potential that both parliamentarians and anthropologists could share some common ground. The advantage of this approach would be that it could take account of what is most central to the parliamentary debates, thus engaging with the mainstream rather than the more refracted vectors. In what remains of this chapter, I have attempted to set out a series of possible analytic approaches to the embryo debates as representations of kinship. To do this, it is first necessary to examine what the parliamentarians have to say about embryos, and to attend to the terms upon which the debate is conducted. This includes the kinds of imagery and metaphor invoked in parliamentary speeches, as well as the kinds of evidence used. By so doing, I would argue, it is possible to identify characteristic features of debate, and thus to pose questions as to why it took the shape it did, what its parameters are and so forth. It is suggested this approach may yield a more effective means of bridging the 'gap' between an anthropological mode of understanding and a parliamentary one.

The embryo debates

If one were an Aristotelian listening to these debates, and asking 'what are they in themselves?', one would have to conclude they are about embryos. In both Second Readings, in the House of Lords and in the House of Commons, nearly all the speakers opened their remarks with facts and opinions about embryos. The Bill itself contained a special drafting innovation to distinguish the embryo question above all else. The main debate preceding parliamentary debate of the Bill was about embryos. It was repeatedly stated that the main question at stake was the embryo question. The formulaic conception recitations were all about the status of the embryo. The embryo question (and, as a consequence, the abortion question)[10] were separated off from the rest of the Bill for debate by a Committee of the Whole House in the Commons. And even the debates of other parts of the Bill can be seen to be marked by politicking aimed at securing gains in relation to the embryo question.[11]

This was true to such an extent as to be remarked upon on more than one occasion. Mary Warnock, for example, no doubt surprised at the extent to which the embryo question overshadowed every other part of the Bill, cautioned against the neglect of other, in her view equally important, issues. Likewise, Lady Saltoun remarked:

> My Lords, I think that everything that can possibly be said about embryo research has already been said over and over again this afternoon and this evening. If one had not seen the Bill and had heard a handful of speeches, one could have been forgiven for being under the impression that it consists of one clause only – Clause 11. Indeed I have spoken to some noble Lords who were under exactly that impression. There is, in fact, quite a lot else in it.
>
> (Lady Saltoun, HL, 7.12.89, c. 1088)

How did the embryo become so central to the Bill? Many of the answers one might provide for this question are inadequate. To say it was because the legislation was drafted in such a way as to make it the main issue only begs the question of why this was so. To say it has implications for abortion is similarly inadequate, as the reason for this is the way the abortion question itself has been framed (in terms of biological facts, fetal personhood, embryo protection and so forth). All indicators point to the 'something special' about the embryo that needs explaining. What would a reading which posits the embryo as a kinship entity reveal?

Debating embryogenesis

> Conception lies at the root of morality.
>
> (Mr Duffy, HC, 23.4.90, c. 57)

In debating embryogenesis, parliamentarians were also debating many other things. Most importantly, they were debating the permissibility, and/ or conditions of permissibility, for embryo research. 'Embryology', part of the Bill's title, is a conflation; it describes *an actual process* of development and *the study of* this process. Debating 'embryology' was therefore an over-determined debate about the future – the future of certain kinds of research, the future of knowledge in this area, the future reproductive possibilities of human beings, the future of human beings yet to be, and the future of legislative measures to regulate all of these future possibilities. As one speaker in the opening debate in the House of Lords put it:

> The Bill is semenal. I apologise for using a word of such ambiguity but it is correct. The Bill is semenal because it is the seed from which all legislation upon the subject will grow. We are at the beginning; at day one, hour one. It behoves us to make sure we have got it right.
>
> (The Earl of Cork and Orrery, HL, 7.12.89, c. 1095)

Such a debate is not only about the future, but also about the past. They are also debating their common origins:

> At one stage in our lives all of us present in this Chamber were indistinguishable little globules made up of a few cells.
>
> (Lord Zuckerman, HL, 7.12.89, c. 1041)

In this respect, the potentiality of the embryo both represents the potentiality of each individual (the future) and is a representation of common ancestry (the past). Its representation in this manner suggests connectedness; all of us are undifferentiated in this respect:

> Whether we choose to play with words about embryos, pre-embryos, fetuses or whatever, every one of us started our lives as an embryo. We should not therefore imagine that what we are talking about is something different from ourselves.
>
> (Sir Michael McNair-Wilson, HC, 23.4.90, c. 89)

The embryo is here described as a universal fact of our shared humanity, which we each embody. The embryo is in this sense also a form of symbolic shared bodily substances, shared *procreative* substance. It carries in it the essence of each individual, a unified 'organising power':

> [A] radical new starting point is provided by the fusion of egg and sperm which introduces *an intrinsic organising power*, independent of further outside stimulus, equipped for the development of full human capacities.
>
> (Lord Harvington, HL, 7.12.89, c. 1070; my emphasis)

> A unique biological event occurs with the conjunction of egg and sperm, as I am sure we will all agree. The contribution of modern genetics has shown ... that the genetic code is a fundamental organising principle and that there is radical unity long before the fourteen-day stage.
>
> (Mr Duffy, HC, 2.4.90, c. 943)

> The potential for a human being lies within the cell to which I have referred. It is as though the computer programme exists, but it has not yet been triggered.
>
> (Mrs Rosie Barnes, HC, 23.4.90, c. 80)

This is why the embryo is 'special': it is connected to us (by its potential to become one of us, just as we were once one of its kind).

In this sense, to debate embryogenesis is to debate humanity itself:

> The word 'conceptus' ... is a good term ... to define the particular period while the chromosomal material from the mother and the father is being reorganised into the potentiality of a new individual. The conceptus can be thought of as a blueprint, and the embryo can be thought of as the individual which results from the blueprint having been achieved ... but the point about using the word 'conceptus' is that in that stage the fertilised egg is a concept of a new individual and not the individual. It is only when the blueprint has been achieved and the building begins – one brick being laid on the next – that one can say the embryo starts.
>
> (Lord Adrian, HL, 6.2.90, c. 725)

The idea of the 'unique genetic blueprint' is not only what makes the embryo special, it has a status in and of itself: 'At conception, the DNA is in place. That is the code of life, and from that moment on it is due respect' (Sir Trevor Skeet, HC, 23.4.90, c. 84).

The embryo not only signifies connectedness in terms of its significance as symbolic procreative substance and its status as a common human origin, it also signifies connectedness metonymically, as a part of our humanity which represents the whole:

> The conclusions we reach about the tiny, vulnerable, powerless human embryo will later shape how we regard the status of every individual and how we perceive his or her human rights. It will determine our attitude towards disabled people, the senile, the incurably sick and the terminally ill. This supreme human rights issue is of the highest moral significance.
>
> (Mr David Alton, HC, 2.4.90, c. 965)

Clearly, this is a Christian position, as indicated by Alton's later comments:

> Concern for the human embryo is part of a seamless garment. That garment is woven together by a common thread. Here is a concern for life, justice, care and worth. When one considers the degradation of life today, destruction of family life, collapse of communities and plunder of creation and indifference to the world's hungry and poor, one can see how that seamless garment has become a tatter of rags. That is what happens when society ceases to believe that each person is unique, *sculpted in the image of his maker*, and not to be treated as expendable raw material. The bill represents a crossroads. . . . I hope the House agrees that to embark on the use of the tiniest human being as the subject of experimentation is a dangerous departure from civilised ways. I say in conclusion to the Hon. Member for Caernarfon [Mr Wigley], who said 'Knock and the door will be opened': 'In as much as ye have done it to the least of these my brethren, ye have done it to me.'
>
> (Mr David Alton, HC, 2.4.90, c. 967, my emphasis)

While the explicit Christian message of this argument might be seen to undermine the perception of the embryo as a kinship entity in the anthropological sense, it should be noted that recognising the embryo as a potential 'brethren', and the analogy between Christian unity and 'society', both presume a basis for recognising the *embryo* as 'one of us'.[12]

Other explicitly Christian speakers make clear that one basis for this recognition of the embryo is secular, by positing that the existence of DNA is what enables it to develop in God's image:

> [F]rom fertilisation onwards the embryo contains its own DNA or

blueprint to enable it to become a unique fully grown person in the image of God and loved by him.

(Lord Robertson, HL, 7.12.89, c. 1093)

What is agreed upon by all is that the embryo is human, it is a being, and 'it has a particular character' (The Lord Bishop of London, HL, 6.3.90, c. 1062). It is for these reasons that the Bill is needed to show proper respect for its status. In this sense, the 'origin' of the Bill itself lies in this need to show respect for embryos. And it is because the embryo needs this recognition that a 'legislative vacuum' was created by its extraction from the womb:

[A] system of legal controls is provided because of *the need to show proper respect to the gametes and human embryos*. . . . Whether or not an embryo is to be treated as a child or a person it clearly has the potential for human life and should be treated with the dignity such status deserves. At present there is a legislative vacuum and it is the duty of Parliament to see that this vacuum is adequately filled.

(The Lord Chancellor, HL, 7.12.89, c. 1011; my emphasis)

As the Secretary of State for Health, Mr Kenneth Clarke, observed in his opening remarks introducing the Commons debate of Clause 11 (concerning embryo research):

Central to the debate is the status which each individual Member will decide, according to his or her own conscience, should rightly be accorded to the embryo. Central to this is the question of when a human comes into existence. . . . The evolution of a human being and citizen from the potential that arises when sperm and egg are first united is a steady and continuous process, and it is difficult to say at what stage a citizen and a human being appears. . . . I think that there is a gulf that cannot be bridged between those who cannot, in all conscience, countenance the idea of research on human embryos, and those who believe that . . . it can be justified. However, there is one small but essential area of common ground – *that there is something special about the human embryo*.

(Mr Clarke, HC, 23.4.90, cols. 33, 34, 41; my emphasis)

From these perspectives, it can be seen that debating embryogenesis formed the 'core' of parliamentary debate. Its centrality was overdetermined, resulting as much from proximate political cause and new technology as from the *longue durée* of Western intellectual fascination with the embryo in terms of science, theology and metaphysics, and much else in between. It is for these reasons that the centrality of the embryo debates to the parliamentary passage of the HFEB is at once obvious and in need of deeper explication. At the very least, I suggest it was pre-eminently in this sphere that representations were being made of a kinship which is 'unfamiliar'.

Kinship trajectories

The explanatory framework which establishes the connectedness between parliamentarians and embryos (as in the 'we were once all tiny globules' argument) is that of biological development. This explanation invokes a particular form of developmental essentialism (teleology), complementing or seen to be manifesting the idea of the 'intrinsic organising power' of the 'genetic blueprint'. The force of this construction of the embryo's (onto-logical) *potential* rests on the assumption that is has *within itself* a particular direction and purpose. Its future form is already written into it: it has a unique design, the design of a potential individual person. This trajectory *(telos)* is integral to the logic enabling parliamentarians to argue about persons-yet-to-be (yet to be even conceived, for that matter) on the basis of their own personal origins. In order for the idea that an embryo is to become what we already are to make sense, a conceptual slippage or substi-tution is required. Hence, along the developmental trajectory – which is continually being debated in terms of whether it is continuous or not – certain substitutions appear. 'All of us here in this chamber' must be substi-tutable for the embryo (or 'pre-embryo') at the two-cell, or eight-cell or fourteen-day stage.

In addition, certain constructions of reproductive time appear in the debate which suggest that the developmental trajectory necessary to the substitution of embryos for adults, and vice versa, *also characterises other kinds of development.* For example, the development of research, science, civilisation, the law, morality and technology are seen to 'follow a similar path'. Or, their paths could be said to share a certain form, characterised by its source (an essential, intrinsic 'organising power') and its direction, which is guided by this inner, unstoppable 'motor' or 'clock'. The development of the embryo has the capacity to stand for both kinds of progress, *indeed to unite them*:

> I am convinced that research and experimentation are a natural part of the development of the human condition. They are almost an essential part of the development of our lives.
>
> (Mr Mallon, HC, 23.4.90, c. 68)

Here, 'embryology', in the sense of the *study* of embryos is seen in almost organic terms, as an 'essential' component of human development. Hence, embryonic development, the study of this process, 'the human condition' and 'the development of our lives' are linked together by a shared, essential developmental trajectory. It is the striking metonymy of these accounts, whereby each developmental trajectory not only 'stands for', but is conflated with, the others which is of note. In sum there is a theme of progress, in its many senses, and particularly in its modernist sense (as a kind of essential truth which is in fact a kind of faith). The definitive feature of this social construction of sequential events in terms of an *intrinsically generated trajectory of progress*, be it organic growth, scientific 'advances' or manifest destiny, is its inevitable emphasis upon the future. Thus, one might consider the following extracts about embryonic development, the development of embryology and reproductive time, simply in terms of *the social construction of sequences*. How are things constructed as sequential, what are the links that make them so, and does this comprise a pattern of cultural logic connecting otherwise disparate domains?

> [T]he subject of our debate is the embryonic human, a living dynamic being having its origin in the meeting of human sperm with the human egg. At the point of fertilisation an irreversible process of human development begins. *It is here that our clock starts.* Before that point new life is a possibility; thereafter, it is an actuality.
>
> (Sir Bernard Braine, HC, 23.4.90, c. 47; my emphasis)

The idea of a starting point is central to several of the subjects that were considered in the debate. It is the means by which continuous processes of development, organic or otherwise, can be broken into sub-sequences, with definitive beginnings. The idea of a starting point, then, is part of the effort to establish limits, boundaries and prohibitions. Of course, at a practical level, this is intended for the purpose of law-making, in order that clear regulations can be established and enforced. However, the parliamentary debate, because it must attend to the justification of such 'lines being drawn', is metaphysical, rather than merely concerned with jurisprudence. As Braine continues: 'What we are being led to legislate for is the beginning' (c. 50). As he has just said: 'We are legislating for the future and for the future of later generations' (c. 47).

An opposing argument, presented by Sir Ian Lloyd in the House of Commons, offers a different picture of what is at stake for future generations. He is concerned with a different 'irreversible process', that of science:

The discovery of DNA, the very blueprint of life, is certainly awe-inspiring, and when the full map of the human genome is known, probably within a decade, we shall have passed through a phase of human civilisation as significant as, if not more significant than, that which distinguished the age of Galileo from that of Copernicus, or that of Einstein from that of Newton. Its political significance is almost beyond our comprehension. We have crossed a boundary of unprecedented importance . . . there is no going back. . . . We are walking hopefully into the scientific foothills of a gigantic mountain range. Hitherto, man has had no option but to come to terms with a serious burden of genetic impairment, but now he can look ahead, perhaps a long way, to its eventual elimination. . . . For us to forswear the assistance which science can provide in modifying that code to the advantage of the human race would be an indefensible abdication of responsibility. It would cross the portcullis of this place with a most sinister and destructive bar.

(Sir Ian Lloyd, HC, 23.4.90, cols. 96–8)

In Lloyd's view, the 'boundary' has already been crossed, we are already in the 'gene age', on a new terrain, in new 'foothills'. There is no stopping this advance, we cannot 'close the doors' on the 'frontiers of human knowledge'; to do so would not only be 'unenforceable', but would 'merely inflame curiosity'. Hence, one essential humanness, the will to know, driven by curiosity and moral purpose, along an unstoppable trajectory of manifest destiny and scientific progress, opposes the view of an essential humanness which demands a respect unconscionably contravened by 'treating it as a guinea pig' or as 'a means to an end'.

The unstoppable force of progress is a reference point for many parliamentarians. As Robert Key observed:

We must come to terms with the inevitable scientific progress. . . . Make no mistake – the work will go on in other countries with or without us. . . . When Parliament or rulers have sought to impose bans on science, or to legislate against progress, they have always come to grief.

(Mr Key, HC, 2.4.90, cols. 953–4)

Many different images surround the debate over the development of embryological knowledge through embryo research. One set of images denotes discontinuity, such as 'threshold', 'watershed', 'rubicon', 'boundary' or 'lines being drawn'. An opposing set of images accompanies the representation of the difficulty of establishing limits. Of these, the two most important are 'the thin end of the wedge' and 'the slippery slope', denoting the inadequacy of proposed regulation to contain the force of the trajectory it seeks to limit:

> If the principle is breached, there is no escaping the consequences. Once one accepts that a human being, *at whatever stage in its development*, can be used for scientific experiment, the rubicon has been crossed and there is no turning back.
>
> (Dame Jill Knight, HC, 2.4.90, c. 957; my emphasis)

This extract demonstrates the idea of substitutability of one stage of human development for another. It is also typical of the kinds of imagery surrounding the debate over 'the way forward'. This is elsewhere described as 'a terrible path', 'the wrong road' and 'the slippery slope'. What is significant about this language is, again, its use across a range of quite different subjects, all of which are constructed as dilemmas in terms of *the difficulty of imposing limits*:

> We have heard a great deal about the slippery slope. I do not subscribe to the view of the slippery slope. Those who believe in it must accept that we are already on the slippery slope, like it or not. The Bill gives us a firm foothold. It gives the public and the scientist the certainty that they want. We must remember that *if we had no Bill we would have no limits*.
>
> (Lord Meston, HL, 7.12.89, c. 1105; my emphasis)

The problem of establishing limits is a problem of 'drawing lines' across what are perceived not only as *continuous* trajectories, but as *internally generated* ones. It is this perception which makes any 'line' appear arbitrary and provisional. Identifying a point of discontinuity along a continuous trajectory evoked different responses. Some parliamentarians saw obvious 'milestones' or 'markers' upon which to base their arguments:

> There is one thing that can be said about the event of conception: before it there is no human being; after it, although not immediately afterwards, there is. It is therefore a milestone between the non-existence of a human being and the existence of a human being. There is a gap between the two, but how big that gap is in my submission does not matter. The moment of conception is the only possible dividing line one can establish.
>
> (The Earl of Cork and Orrery, HL, 7.12.89, c. 1095)

The opposing view was put forward by Lord Walton:

> [C]onception is not a moment in time but a process in time. . . . In our ordinary lives, we are not accustomed to processes which have no definable or identifiable beginning. . . . There is an identifiable beginning to one's terminal illness. . . . The process of fertilisation is something which has no identifiable beginning. . . . The process of penetration is not like sticking a drawing pin into a piece of paper.
>
> (Lord Walton, HL, 6.2.90, c. 724)

Despite these differences, certain shared recognitions characterise the parliamentary debates about embryogenesis. The 'special' character of the embryo is recognised as its 'genetic blueprint' which is seen as the source of its developmental potential. The blueprint *is* the continuity of the embryo. It is recognised that either the moment when this genetic blueprint is established (although there was debate about whether there was such a moment), or some time along the path of the embryo's subsequent development, a marker had to be found upon which to base legislation. This marker in the end was the emergence of the primitive streak, although, as has already been noted, its actual emergence was not the actual marker. In any event, the source of confusion seems partly to lie in the way the agreed-upon trajectory of embryogenesis was conceived. If it is seen to contain an intrinsic source of its own continuity, its potential for biological growth, nothing *but* its subsequent development could serve as a basis for a 'marker'. This dilemma was, in fact, never resolved; it was simply superseded by the imposition of a time-limit of fourteen days, justified on the basis of a natural fact it simultaneously rendered irrelevant.

Another dilemma produced by this manner of conceptualising the developmental trajectory of the embryo was that already mentioned at the outset of this section: the conceptual substitutability of one stage of human development for another. Several parliamentary speakers employed this as a mode of reasoning: 'We regard the embryo as a born child or a grown up,' stated the Duke of Norfolk on behalf of the parliamentary Pro-Life group (HL, 6.2.90, c. 746). Baroness Elles added that:

> Fertilisation is the start of a process of growth and development which through childhood produces an adult human being. As the Warnock Report states, no particular part of the development and process is more important than any other; all are part of a continuous process.
>
> (Baroness Elles, HL, 6.2.90, c. 716)

Perhaps both the conflation of stages along this trajectory and the problem of demarcating its continuity at any stage comes from its non-relational constitution. Having constructed a completely genetic basis for personhood, which is also the essence of the trajectory (the realisation of the genetic blueprint), the parliamentarians were left with a closed circuit. In one of the few effective challenges to this construction of embryo-genesis, it was left to the Archbishop of York to break into the sanctum of the embryo's protected and essential individuality by asserting its relatedness:

> The argument is constantly made that such a conceptus might develop into one of us. Indeed there is a great difference between reading history backwards and trying to predict it forwards. When you read history backwards you can trace out a train of cause and event; you can trace back an individual life in which we rejoice now to its earliest beginnings *in the womb and beyond in the life of its parents.* However, when you are trying to read history forwards you are simply talking of potentialities. What we are talking about when we look at a conceptus is a potential for life. *Unless that conceptus is actually implanted in a uterus* it has no potential beyond those few days during which experimentation takes place. . . . Nobody in their wildest dreams would want to say that infanticide is justified if research on a conceptus is justified. That is to ignore the whole process which has taken place in between.
> (The Archbishop of York, HL, 8.2.90, c. 956; my emphasis)

The assumption that the embryo has within it a genetic blueprint, the making of its own future, as well as the information about the unique individual it will become, is the basis for the substitutability of different stages of development here criticised by the Archbishop of York – that one stage can be thought of in terms of a subsequent stage. His point, that the embryo's development is not purely individual, and his reference to its relational character, immediately invoked its social context. The fact that the embryo is dependent upon its mother to develop was also stated by MP Audrey Wise:

> The long title of the Bill says that the Act will 'make provision in connection with human embryos and any subsequent development of such embryos' which is a strange and rather sweeping statement. *We are all, after all, the subsequent development of embryos* and I wondered how far this matter might go. . . . If we are to deal with fetuses in the Bill, why cannot we deal with, for example, the proper nourishment of expectant mothers? . . . Why cannot I table amendments to deal with social security matters to put these problems right? . . . If the House

were so interested in the welfare of children, many women would not feel the desperation that drives them to seek abortions. . . . The embryo is not a human being. In an ectopic pregnancy the embryo cannot develop into a human being. . . it is not in itself a human being, [it] cannot be regarded as such. . . . There has been a good deal of hypocrisy in this debate.

(Mrs Audrey Wise, HC, 2.4.90, c. 974; my emphasis)

Such a statement embeds embryonic development not only in relation to the mother (more commonly referred to as the embryo's 'source of nutrition' or its 'environment'), but in relation to society. Here, the microscopic lens of embryology is extended, relationally, to encompass *the social context of the embryo*, a perspective that is muted in the debates as a whole. It creates the perspective familiar to anthropologists in their dealings with kinship. But such statements were exceptional. To understand more fully how the terms of the embryo debates were shaped, the next section examines the use of evidence in order to suggest that the whole debate was about, among other things, the construction and negotiation of unfamiliar kinship.

THE USE OF EVIDENCE

As there are well-established conventions of parliamentary discourse, it is safe to assume that even in a debate as admittedly unusual as that surrounding the passage of the HFEA, many forms of speech or argument are unacceptable and inappropriate. Of these conventions, the most often remarked upon are emotional language, inappropriate accusations, and disorderly behaviour. Even so, the kinds of evidence mustered by parliamentarians on either side of the embryo question were circumscribed. Indeed, all the evidence could be grouped into four categories. The most prominently cited source of evidence was that of the established experts, including various professional groups, such as doctors, lawyers, academics, theologians and, most importantly, scientists. A second category of evidence had been provided by voluntary organisations and charities, such as infertility and handicap support groups. There were then two categories of 'affected persons': the experienced parents (especially 'mums') of genetically handicapped children, and the infertile couples or couples with a high risk of passing on severe genetic disorders.

The first two categories represent expert opinion, based on criteria regarded as objective, such as research or 'facts and figures', mostly from specialists in the area. The second two categories rely on a different 'truth', that of experience. These two groups also represented different kinds of 'pleas' to parliamentarians. In the former case, the aim was to provide better care, services or health provision, on behalf of others. In the second category, the aim was to improve one's own lot or, if not to alleviate one's own suffering, to see improvements in the lives of others who shared one's plight.

Parliamentarians employed this evidence in a variety of ways. They quoted from newspaper articles, surveys, books, speeches and various other published sources. They read extracts from correspondence, either from affected constituents or influential experts who sent them information. They described particular cases, or cited particular instances as demonstrating their point. They referred to government documents and legislation, as well as the *Official Record*, and often to legislation in other countries. Finally, they occasionally made reference to their own personal experience. This was nearly always in the context of their professional work, but sometimes involved the use of personal anecdote or, more rarely, personal kinship ties. For example, a handful of parliamentarians either had disabled children, had undergone infertility treatment or, in two cases, had seen their own children die from severe congenital disorders.

This final section is devoted particularly to the kinship evidence presented by various speakers. This is the one dimension of the debates where relationships *were* brought in as evidence in support of arguments. The way relationships were represented, however, tended to be formulaic. The conventions of this mode of representation were therefore revealing not only in terms of what they included, but what they left out. As will become evident, this form of the representation of kinship in the context of NRTs reveals a novel character indeed.

Among the conventions through which parliamentarians position themselves as speakers in debate is the manner of introducing statements with a disclaimer: the speaker begins by signalling lack of expertise, particularly (in this debate) scientific expertise. This took the form of 'I am not a scientist/ theologian/other expert, but . . .', and little affected their subsequent remarks. Parliamentarians are also required to declare any interests which might be seen to influence their opinions, and thus, members of the Royal Society, the Medical Research Council and so forth, would duly declare their membership of these bodies at the outset of their speeches. In the case of theological positions, a declaration of religious affiliation explicitly established the speaker's perspective as a point of view they brought to the debate.

Disclaimers were sometimes employed in relation to the kinship position of the speaker. For example, in the opening debate of the Bill, in the Second Reading in the House of Lords, Baroness Elles stated:

My Lords, it is only in your Lordships' House that one could ever have the privilege of hearing a debate such as we have heard tonight. Many distinguished theologians, our noble and learned friend the Lord Chancellor and many distinguished scientists have taken part. It is therefore perhaps appropriate, as one of the few here tonight, that I should speak as a simple mother and grandmother. After all, we are talking about children and births.

(Baroness Elles, HL, 7.12.89, c. 1075)

This extract usefully exemplifies several aspects of the formulaic disclaimer. In highlighting scientific and theological expertise, it accurately reflects the consistent priority afforded these two forms of expertise in the debate as whole. Second, in its praise for the parliamentary process, it is also typical, for such polite pronouncements are frequently encountered at the outset of speeches, acting as a kind of framing device or refrain in debate. The contrast between the conventional forms of address such as 'distinguished', 'noble' and 'learned' to describe scientists, theologians and parliamentarians, and the almost self-deprecating adjective 'simple' to describe her own 'expertise' as a mother, is pronounced. In its reference to the exclusion of women, the experience of motherhood and 'maternal knowledge' from debate, an exclusion which occurs to the most profound degree, it simultaneously makes reference to the *obvious* significance of this perspective: '*After all*, we are talking about children and births'. One might suggest it is therefore an explicit reference to a shared relational experience among parliamentarians, which elsewhere acts as an implicit sub-text, though such a claim would be difficult to establish.[13]

In a statement shortly afterwards, the Baroness continued:

Again, I speak as a parent, I myself was fortunate to have healthy children. However we all know many parents who have not. The other night I was talking to a friend and said how fortunate I was and that I would speak with great humility in this debate. I was asked what I was going to say and I replied roughly that I had had the good fortune to have healthy children. He said, 'Don't worry, I have a child who has Down's syndrome and I cannot tell you how happy I am to have had that child.' I think we must sometimes remember that love of one's child, with all its human defects – whether physical or mental – plays a far greater role than has so far been touched upon.

(Baroness Elles, HL, 7.12.89, c. 1076)

In so far as it directly addresses an ambivalence about the experiences of parents with handicapped children, and the feelings of those who have 'healthy' children in relation to these parents, this extract is exemplary of the character of the debates as a whole. But it is also explicit in its identification of an absence in the debate, of a silence around actual relationships, such as those between parents and children. It locates the speaker in a very personal way; as soon as a kinship position, a relational position, is established, it becomes possible to speak in a different tenor, openly expressing deeply felt concerns through a narrative testimonial based on personal experience. Speaking 'as a parent' or as a 'simple mother and grandmother' enables a different form of address; it proposes an utterly different terrain from that of noble and distinguished scientists speaking with the certainty of their authoritative expertise.

The Baroness's reference to parents of handicapped children is to be understood in relation to the tremendous importance accorded to these parents and to the experience of infertile couples in debate. The main argument concerning these couples was that science could help them have healthy children and that Parliament must not close the door on their only source of hope. These parents, it was argued, have a right to the choices made available to them by modern science, and there was a duty for Parliament to uphold this right. As Lord Ennals argued:

> We are embarking on the consideration of a Bill that will profoundly affect the lives and the hopes of thousands of families now and in the future . . . . We are talking about research which could be of great potential to humanity. Its prohibition could cause great sadness, pain and suffering and end the hopes of many hard-pressed and worried families, not only now but also in the future . . . . The case I wish to make is the right to choose . . . it cannot be right for people not directly or personally affected by the issues involved to deny the benefits of carefully controlled, inspected and limited research to people troubled by infertility or those concerned about the avoidance of physical and mental handicap.
>
> (Lord Ennals, HL, 7.12.89, c. 1012)

Two features of this extract particularly elucidate the general character of parliamentary debate on this subject. The first is the emphasis upon the right to choose the benefits of scientific progress. If the (developmental) potential of the early embryo is, for the opponents of embryo research, its metonymic potential to stand for the whole of humanity, then here the opposite picture is depicted. In this view, it is not the *embryo* but the potential of embryo *research* which stands for collective humanity: 'the great potential for humanity'. The contrast is between embryo*genesis* and embry*ology*. But the second point is equally important. There is also a different thread of individualism at the root of this argument. Again, it is not the essential, definitive individuality of the embryo, it is the alternative, humanist individualism of *the right to choose*. This leads us to a most important point about evidence: 'It cannot be right *for people not directly or personally affected by the issues involved* to deny the benefits [to others who are].' This is also an argument about *individual experience* and *individual desires.*

This argument introduces the importance of the case study and the visit to the clinic, two frequently used forms of evidence. The argument is that if one does not agree with embryo research, one simply need not partake in its benefits, and must not on such grounds deny them to others. It is *these significant others* to whom the advocates of this position point again and again: to those people who are 'directly and personally affected'. The opponents of this view, who argue that the embryo is part of a shared humanity, and that how it is treated therefore affects *all* of us, whether we use the benefits of embryo research or not, *have nothing to point to but the embryo itself.* This, in addition to the fact that despite science and theology being the two privileged forms of expertise, they are privileged unequally – science being seen as neutral and theology being seen as a particular point of view (e.g. Catholic, Methodist, Jewish, Anglican) – disadvantaged the anti-embryo-research parliamentarians considerably.

A few examples of the prominence given to the evidence of childless couples and carriers of genetic diseases will suffice. Though they are ubiquitous throughout the debates, it is striking that, like the media representations of the 'desperate' infertile couple, they are formulaic in their adherence to readily identifiable, and quite narrow, representational parameters.[14] One might say they were in this sense generic:

> Some women have seen their brothers, nephews and uncles die of dreadful diseases that affect only the males in their families. They may have a child already afflicted by the same disease, or they may have had a late abortion, having discovered at 19 or 20 weeks that they were carrying a boy child. Should we condemn those women to childlessness? . . . Women such as myself who have had children fairly easily find it difficult to comprehend the misery of childlessness. However, if one talks to someone who has been trying to have a child for 10 years or more and who watches sisters, and even her nieces and friends producing children and who feels inadequate and unfulfilled and less than a woman, one begins to understand the pain and misery. We must continue to recognise and tackle the problem.
>
> (Mrs Rosie Barnes, HC, 23.4.90, cols. 80–1)

In outlining the plight of the two main categories of affected persons, this extract illustrates the generic conventions structuring the use of evidence.

A variant on this personal witness approach is the professional witness:

> Here I must declare an interest as current chairman of the Muscular Dystrophy Group of Great Britain and Northern Ireland. . . . As I became immersed in that work, I became increasingly concerned and deeply affected by the plight of patients with that disease and by the immense burden of care which it imposed upon their families. As one mother said poignantly: 'I see my son die a little every day.'
>
> (Lord Walton, HL, 7.12.89, c. 1052)

Here a direct quotation establishes the testimony of 'an affected person'. This evidence relied on a form of truth recognised by the speakers as different from that of the scientific fact. It was not concerned with objective natural facts but with subjective social facts. It rests on the authority of experience, and upon the ability of parliamentarians to identify with this. Indeed, opposing parliamentarians were often at pains to demonstrate their sympathy for the sufferers of infertility and genetic disorders before going on to argue that even so they could not countenance embryo research. At times they were explicitly critical of this form of argument:

> The joy of those who achieve fertility or are able to achieve a baby through IVF has been described from all sides of the House. It is developing a special place in this argument.
>
> (Lord Kennet, HL, 7.12.89, c. 1028)

This recognition of the 'special place' accorded to this form of evidence acknowledges the key role it played in the debate as a whole. Emotive, often graphic, and of invariably tragic proportions, the spotlighting of case studies, including those of some parliamentarians themselves, was discomfortingly, and accurately, perceived by opponents of embryo research as having a near unanswerable status in debate for reasons that were obvious but also worrying.

Yet, answer such examples they did. Not only was the 'special place' of such arguments challenged, but they were challenged with counter-examples and by reasoned argument. For example, they were challenged by speakers who pointed out that just because someone has the experience of being infertile or of carrying a severe genetic disease does not necessarily mean such persons take scientific research on embryos to be a good thing. Bernard Braine read out letter from an infertile couple who were 'anxious to correct the seriously misleading impression that human embryo experimentation is necessary for people like us' (HC, 23.4.90, c. 49). In a similar counter-argument, Dame Jill Knight spoke in the House of Lords of her own experience of losing a congenitally disabled child while still remaining in opposition to embryo research. The opposite position was argued by Daffydd Wigley, in the House of Commons, who movingly spoke of the death of his two sons from genetically inherited abnormalities and his own support of embryo research. Unlike objective scientific facts, which are simply 'true' and accepted as such, even if they are partial or poorly understood, the truth of experience is constructed as individual and personal. It relies not on the acceptance of the listener, but on their ability to identify with it in relation to their own experiences. It is in this double sense a relational form of truth.

Finally there was the visit to the clinic. This was said to have influenced several parliamentarians' decision-making processes. Arrangements had been made, by Lord Jellicoe, a member of the House of Lords and the Medical Research Council, with a number of clinics to enable parliamentarians to visit their premises and 'see for themselves' the work that was being done. Here they were able to meet clinicians and patients, and to observe the techniques involved if they so chose. For parliamentarians such as Baroness Llewelyn-Davies, the experience of visiting a clinic proved decisive:

> IVF has seemed almost like a miracle for desperately unhappy childless couples who are able to undertake the new process. . . . I am speaking today because I have been able to visit the IVF clinic at Addenbrookes Hospital in Cambridge. . . . I saw one woman who is a senior midwife. She loves her work and is obviously dedicated to her patients, but until now she has had the experience of delivering babies day by day while unable to have one of her own. She has had two failed IVF pregnancies but is now in the 25th week of her third pregnancy and is expecting twins, if all goes well. She has to stay in bed in the clinic for a highly critical period of time just now, and probably for most of the rest of her pregnancy, but she said: 'It's all worth it – without IVF I would never have had the chance of having a child.'
>
> (Baroness Llewelyn-Davies, HL, 7.12.89, cols. 1023–4)

In the representation of the visit to the clinic and the case study are combined two types of testimonial: that of the parliamentarian and that of the affected person. Thus, the parliamentarian is describing her or his own personal experience of someone else's personal experience, and by so doing making a formal, public declaration and a formal public record of the domain of the personal, which is then complemented by other, more authoritative, kinds of facts and knowledge.

The conventions of this form of representation demonstrate an interesting feature of this kind of evidence: like the embryo debate, it is about potentialities. This evidence is about the *desire* to *become* a parent. It is about children yet to be. It is about the *potential* for research to help people. The only reference to *actual* relationships is in cases where the families of afflicted children are described. In such representations are brought together all of the potentialities discussed earlier with respect to the embryo debates: the potential of scientific research; of technological enablement; and of new 'relations', in terms of both new persons and new ties.

This returns us to the extract from Baroness Elles's speech at the opening of this section (p. 153). The ambivalence she describes towards the experience of parents with handicapped children runs through the debate. On the one hand, the aim of enabling parents who are at risk of producing children with genetic handicaps is held up as a reason for promoting research, to eliminate handicap. Yet, there is also the wish to acknowledge that handicapped children are not simply a burden to their parents, but may create as much, or even more, joy as healthy children. In other words, in the only case where actual relationships are referred to, the matter is somewhat blurred. It is in the cases where *a relationship does not yet exist*, where parents feel they cannot have children because they are carriers of severe genetic abnormalities, or simply cannot have children at all because they are infertile, that the matter is clear-cut.

But of what does such evidence consist? As Lord Ennals said, it consists of 'the lives and hopes of thousands of families now *and in the future*'. It is so that couples can 'enjoy marriages in which they can *look forward* to producing children free of such dreadful diseases' (Mr Thurnham, HC, 23.4.90, c. 62; my emphasis). It is 'to promote *the generation of life* for those who would otherwise be infertile' (Lord Jakobovits, HL, 7.12.89, c. 1072; my emphasis). The evidence presented, the *only* evidence which *would* be about kinship relationships is, in fact, about kinship *potentials*, future kinship trajectories which, as yet, exist only in the form of desires and the right to choose. This 'kinship' is about families, relationships, parents and children, which do not yet exist. Hence, although 'relationships' were represented, it was in the service of arguing for potential relationships yet to be. Indeed, it was not really about relationships at all, but rather the potential for *science and technology* to bring them into being, to bring new and improved kinds of persons, families and relationships into being.

CONCLUSION: WHAT KIND OF KINSHIP?

> [R]esearch can be beneficial to humankind . . . it can be creative rather
> than destructive. Some of that research will not bear fruit for many
> years, perhaps not until we in this House have retired or passed on.
> Therefore, we are legislating for the future and for the future of later
> generations.
>
> (Ms Jo Richardson, HC, 23.4.90, c. 47)

What was the character of the 'kinship' that was being debated by parliamentarians? This chapter has contrasted two ways in which we might make sense of this character. In the first section, 'Familiar kinship', the representation of kinship in the context of parliamentary debate is analysed according to approaches that are conventional and well established within anthropology. From this vantage point, the negotiation of kinship contained in the parliamentary speeches have analogues in other cultures, as in the redefinition of the relationship between social and natural facts in the context of discussions of conception and the origin of persons. From this perspective, ethnographic comparison reduces the apparent novelty of contemporary concerns so that they appear more familiar, conventional, indeed even traditional. Such a perspective necessarily relies upon and also confirms, a traditional anthropological expertise concerning kinship.

An alternative approach is suggested in the second section of this chapter, 'Unfamiliar kinship', which attempts to address some of the features of parliamentary debate which do not fit as easily into established anthropological frameworks. Here, emphasis is placed upon the centrality of the individuated, non-relational embryo to these debates. I have suggested this is an 'unfamiliar' kinship entity warranting closer interrogation.

By positing the embryo as an unfamiliar kinship entity, or as a condensed symbolic signifier of an unfamiliar kind of kinship, my aim is both to make new kinds of 'kinship' visible, and to question what is meant by the concept. If we rewrite their concerns as an attempt to elucidate the foundations of kinship in contemporary culture, then some of the parliamentarians' dilemmas become shared with those of the anthropologist. Though not incompatible with more established anthropological understandings of kinship, such an approach might in turn refract upon, and refigure them.

In the third section, 'The use of evidence', an attempt is made to consolidate this approach through analysis of the representation of kinship relations in parliamentary debate. Building on the evidence provided in the earlier two sections, the third section illustrates the character of kinship emergent in the context of new reproductive technologies. In the remainder of this chapter, then, is a summary of what this 'unfamiliar kinship' may be seen to comprise.

What kind of kinship is this?

Most evident in the preceding section, and underscored by the headnote to the conclusion, is the extent to which the representation of kinship relations in parliamentary debate is structured around *potentials*. In this sense, the strikingly non-relational character of kinship debate is in part explained by its preoccupations with *kinship yet-to-be* or *future kinship*. As we have seen, there are several potentialities at stake, not just future researches, future relationships and future persons but the future implications of all of these, extending from their impact upon particular individuals to their meaning for society, morality and humanity in general.

The 'kinship' represented in the parliamentary debates is one in which, in addition to social facts and natural facts, a third order of facts has come to be paramount: those of science and technology. The evidence for this new foundation of kinship extends from the title of the Bill to the privileging of scientific expertise in the debate to the treatment of the embryo as a 'cult object', as Lord Kennet described it. If so, then the embryo *embodies* this foundation. It is not only a 'new' kind of kinship entity, in the sense of requiring clarification of its relational status, but the embodiment of a 'new' kind of kinship, in its embodiment of scientific progress and technological potency.

The fact of having been brought into being by technology also determines the nature of the embryo as kinship entity. The new kinship is one that can be controlled from within: it is not only assisted nature, it is nature redesigned. It is a nature that *requires* intervention, as well as legal clarification, in order to express itself. Its 'literal message', in the form of the genetic code, is being mapped in order that natural science can rewrite natural fact. Nature is not only 'culturally constructed', it is being physically (re)constructed too. This embryo does not so much embody nature as scientific progress.

It may not be novel to those versed in cross-cultural comparisons to note, as does Rivière, that the social facts of kinship do not match the natural facts of genetic connection. What *is* novel is that the resultant kinships will embody this intervention; that is, these persons will have been physically and morally enabled to come into existence by virtue of the conjoining of science, technology and the law. Just as the birth of Louise Brown embodies the embryo created in vitro by Edwards and Steptoe, just as she embodies the technique itself (her body itself making manifest its potency), just as her birth also brought into being a 'legislative vacuum' that needed to be filled, *so future children will embody the Bill which enabled them to be born*. This is a reproductive cycle in a novel sense. A child is technologically conceived who embodies the need for a law; a law is brought into being because of this child's birth; the law will bring into being other children who will embody it.

Just as the law will bring into being other children, so too will it bring into being forms of 'scientific progress' whose 'fruit' is as yet unknown, the political (and social and cultural) consequences of which are 'almost beyond our comprehension', to quote Ian Lloyd again. What is this almost unthinkable kinship?

There are several possible implications which would need to be explored. What does it mean to point to the desire for children and call it kinship? *Is* it kinship? What are the implications of kinship being rewritten on the terrain of embryology? Is *this* kinship?

If what is most recognisable to anthropologists as kinship does not have much importance to the debate, perhaps we do need to rethink what we recognise as kinship. Grounds for such rethinking already exist within anthropology itself. Specifically, the proposal by Collier and Yanagisako (1987) that it is 'the biological facts of sexual reproduction' which most need explaining in the study of kinship systems would appear highly relevant to the parliamentary debate. Embryology is all about these facts. Kinship in the context of embryology might indeed look unfamiliar. It is micro-kinship, composed of unfamiliar kinship entities, germinal matter in need of classification, symbolic shared procreative substance, a new human 'ancestor'. It is also geneticised, in a symbolic reductionism effecting a simultaneous cellularisation of our origins, identities and inheritances while also making of kinship a universal human connectedness that looks more like the 'family of man'. The new kinship chart is the map of the genome; our shared bodily substance can be banked, patented and protected by antitrust legislation. New kinship boundaries thus emerge. They are not between different families or even between different cultures, but between humans and other species. This is species endogamy. It is structured by a reversed incest taboo, whereby distance, rather than proximity, of relations define procreative proscriptions.[15]

In addition to being technologised and geneticised, the new kinship is also highly individualised. Kinship, in the sense of genetic identity, is seen as essential to the individual. This, too, effects a particular type of reduction-ism. There is no 'genetic identity' without the individual in whom it is manifested, and there is no individuality without genetic identity. So totalis-ing is the individuality of the embryo that even the mother may be rendered invisible. A parallel individualism attends the justification of new repro-ductive technologies in the name of individual desires, rights and choices.

In both instances, a reproductive cycle, like that attending technology, emerges. New individuals are (re)produced in the name of individual rights and choice. Individual rights and choice are realised through the (re)production of new individuals. It is from this individualised discourse that future kinship will issue forth, and so on.

If this is the rewriting of kinship *through a (single) kinship entity*, the embryo, it creates a new kinship difficult to recognise from the vantage point of anthropology. Rewritten through the embryo, itself a discursive product of embryology, kinship is restructured, to say the least. The possibility that both anthropologists *and* parliamentarians are on unfamiliar territory in terms of what is meant by 'kinship' or its foundations raises an intriguing question. In order to explore this question further, we would have to return to anthropology itself to rework our understandings of kinship. And if this makes the task seem much larger, it at least provides a different starting point from which the dilemmas faced by parliamentarians may be better appreciated.

This study began with the assumption that new reproductive technologies not only create new persons, but new relations, in both senses of the term. It is here possible to add that the NRTs not only create new conceptions in the procreative sense, but in the cultural or imaginative sense as well. Not only are new individuals conceived, but new conceptions of kinship and relations are also 'born'. These new ways of 'thinking kinship' may be derivative of new ways of 'doing' procreation, but are not restricted to the domain of assisted reproduction. With assistance to conception comes also assisted origins, assisted relations, assisted genealogy and assisted futures. The meaning of such assistance is not merely additive: it is transformative. One does not only derive new relations, but new ways of understanding relatedness, new implications of relatedness, new joys of relatedness, and new fears about the dangers of relatedness, or of bringing new relations into being.

It is for this reason that a sense of loss, threat and anxiety is so often palpable in the parliamentary debate, as in public discourse more widely, and as frequently encountered in even the most superficial of encounters with the subject of new reproductive technologies. On offer is the realisation of collective hope in the betterment of the human condition through the embodiment of scientific progress. In question are the implications of such progress, indeed whether it is progress at all. The problem for both parliamentarians and anthropologists is that the NRTs not only produce new dilemmas, but also challenge the very terms upon which such dilemmas are understood. How is one to measure consequences that are 'almost beyond our comprehension'?

Unlike the anthropological observer, faced with uncertainty, the parliamentarians were faced by a need for certainty: for guidelines, boundaries, facts, definitions, and above all *limits*. Like nature, society will not tolerate a vacuum. Parliament has succeeded in its aim, by enacting laws, to fill the 'legislative vacuum' surrounding embryos. Yet by so doing, the vacuum is not dissipated, and instead proliferates. It is not, after all, the embryo, but the *assistance to* the embryo which created the vacuum to begin with. And it is this assistance which is legalised by the Act itself. In the end, it is not the embryo, but scientific progress which requires regulation. It is only because the assisted embryo *embodies* this *potential* that it became the focus of debate.

From a speculative entity in the seventeenth century, the modern embryo has emerged as a scientific fact of embryology. Successfully extracted from the 'dark continent' of the maternal body, or created in the petri dish, it has emerged as an 'individual' in the late twentieth century. From a legal nonentity, it has become a civil subject, accorded the attention and respect of parliamentarians and the protection of the state. Clearly, these changes in the meaning of the embryo cannot be separated from the wider social relations which accord it particular conventions of recognition.

Composed of shared bodily substance resulting from procreation, and at the same time making manifest an unprecedented embodiment of scientific progress, the embryo is symbolically overdetermined.[16] Its acquisition of a kinship identity is similarly weighted. If the importance of kinship study to anthropology lies in its interest in the way relations are governed by how we conceptualise them, 'kinship' is a matter of how such relations are 'conceived', and the importance of the embryo as a kinship entity is self-evident. By so concluding, one is both removed from and simultaneously returned to earlier precepts: by reading the embryo as not only constituted by, but constitutive of, the social field surrounding it, a significance to kinship study more characteristic of earlier anthropological eras is revived. So, too, are other anthropological traditions refigured, such as the definition of kinship itself. It is at the point of interplay between these two contrasting perspectives, through which anthropology is thrown back on its own discursive technologies for 'making sense', that a precise parallel with legislating embryology can be drawn.

NOTES

1 For a guide to the Human Fertilisation and Embryology Act, see Morgan and Lee (1991).

2 It should be noted that the centrality of the embryo to parliamentary debate was due in part to its relation to the question of abortion. However, this relation is the product of the abortion question being framed with reference

to the embryo in a manner which itself requires explanation, and is not unrelated to the discussion presented here. Abortion was brought under the remit of the HFEB as a result of purported dissatisfaction with the resolution of parliamentary debate of the Alton Bill in the previous parliamentary session. The Alton Bill, a Private Member's Bill aimed at lowering the upper time limit of abortion, was 'talked out' of Parliament, despite having won a wide measure of support. Hence, it was the decision of the government to include a vote on abortion within the HFEB (see further, Morgan and Lee 1991).

3 Readers with an interest in this debate will find in the Second Reading of the House of Lords a useful summary of many of the most important arguments presented over the subsequent nine months of debate. It is in many ways the heart of the debate in this respect, comprising the initial laying-out of the positions which were to determine the shape of later debates, and in this sense setting the terms for the debate as a whole.

4 For a comparison with debates in other cultures, see Rivière (1985). For an introduction to anthropological debates about conception beliefs, see Montagu (1937) and Delaney (1986); for a review of the history of embryology in this culture, and debates about the nature and meaning of conception, see Needham (1959); for a review of debates within anthropology concerning kinship theory, see Schneider (1984), Gellner (1987).

5 For a discussion of the neglect of kinship studies in contemporary Euro-American culture, and a recent contribution to these, see Strathern (1992a).

6 Difficulties likely to be faced by future parliamentarians were already in the making at the time of the initial debate of the HFEB. In the same month that Parliament began consideration of the HFEB (November 1989), the British government commissioned a Committee of Inquiry into the Ethics of [Human] Gene Therapy, headed by Sir Cecil Clothier. The Report of this Commission, published in January of 1992 (Cm. 1788), just over a year after enactment of the Act, is but one of several forthcoming legislative issues concerning technological assistance to the procreative process.

7 For anthropological studies of new reproductive technologies and related issues outside the UK, see Stolcke (1986), Ginsburg (1989), Rapp (1987, 1995).

8 For an introduction to the debates concerning 'virgin birth' in anthropology, see Malinowski (1927, 1930), Montagu (1937), Leach (1966), Spiro (1965).

9 For an outline of the key 'natural facts' of embryogenesis considered to be the objective, factual basis of state-of-the-art embryology, see Braude and Johnson in Dunstan (1990).

10 See note 2 above.

11 The 'overdeterminedness' of the embryo question can be summarised as its capacity to embody the union of science and nature. See further at note 16 below.

12 The status of the embryo has a long and distinguished history in theological and metaphysical debate. Aristotle's work on generation was the source of many of his theories of causality and form, which via their influence on Sir Thomas Aquinas continue to be a reference point for theological debates today (see Ford 1988). In this sense, the embryo question is far from 'new'.

13 It is more accurate to note the selective inclusion of 'women's interests' in

parliamentary debate than to declare their omission. However, the fore-grounding of the interests of 'desperate' infertile women, as if these technologies were purely beneficial to women, is disingenuous. The harmful effects of NRTs for women who use them, and for women's status in general, is the subject of a considerable feminist literature. Most importantly, the granting of civil rights to the embryo has direct consequences for women's rights and status, most immediately in terms of access to abortion. It creates the situation of two 'individuals' with competing 'rights' inhabiting the same body, thus undermining the concept of 'individual rights', and confounding the Lockean doctrine of 'property in one's person' intrinsic to the ethos of liberal humanism (see further, Franklin, 1991).

14 The representation of 'desperate' couples in need of natural science to achieve a 'natural' family has become a well-known theme in popular media accounts of the new reproductive, and now the new genetic, technologies. For an analysis of the former, see Franklin (1990).

15 Like many taboos, this one has already been broken in the parliamentary decision to permit the so-called 'hamster test', whereby a hamster egg is used to test the ability of weak sperm to penetrate an egg. Since the hamster egg, unusually, if not uniquely, has a removeable zona pellucida (outer layer), it is seen as an irreplaceable component of this test. The assumption is such a union would not be viable, even if it were not destroyed, which is standard procedure. None the less, this test created much unrest among parliamentarians who argued a question of principle was at stake. As in the case of the permissibility of embryo research, the hamster test was seen as a necessary instrument of scientific progress.

16 In its ability to embody the union of science and nature, the embryo might be described as a cyborg kinship entity. In its consequent 'displacement' of previous, foundational assumptions about nature, however, this kinship might also be described as postmodern. Other features of the 'new' kinship might also be described as postmodern, in particular the sense of loss and uncertainty accompanying the endorsement of embryo research in the name of scientific progress, and the doubt felt towards this 'progress' in the very act of endorsing it. To the extent that postmodernism describes a *condition* characterised by loss of legitimacy and foundational authority, accompanied by self-consciousness of doubt and uncertainty where a more convincing set of beliefs or faiths once existed, many of the phenomena described here could be described as symptomatic, or even constitutive of, the condition of postmodernity.

Afterword for Chapter 4
'Orphaned' embryos

Sarah Franklin

In devising legislation to regulate the use of assisted conception technologies over the course of the 1980s, the overriding concern for British parliamentarians was the necessity to establish limits on embryo research. That there is 'something special' about human embryos, and that there must be limits to what can be done to them, were two of the most consistent points of consensus throughout a debate characterised by a widely diverse and passionately contested range of views. Specifying precise limits to embryo research proved a lengthy and exhaustive parliamentary process. Yet, not only were such limits agreed upon, but the enactment of the Human Fertilisation and Embryology Bill in Britain in 1990 established one of the most substantial legislative precedents achieved anywhere in the world in the politically fraught, scientifically complex and uniquely emotive area of new reproductive technologies (NRTs).[1]

One component of this story which will be particularly obvious to anthropologists is that it is, like all reproductive dilemmas, exponential: the very limits set with one hand will no sooner be in place than they are readjusted by the other. How very like a kinship system this narrative must be! For no sooner is a limit established than the very contexts of comparison it enables are undone by the nature of comparison itself: to set one thing against another is to make of any anchor a triangulation to another point of departure.

Before resorting to the position that it is in the nature of any society or its government always to be in the process of resolving its own contradictions, it is useful to consider a specific example. *Plus ça change* may be the refrain, but the details are never irrelevant. Hence, a case in point.

The most prominent limit, the foundational and most symbolic limit point of the Human Fertilisation and Embryology Act, is the fourteen-day restriction on embryo research. This limit emerged as a symbol for the idea of limit itself by simple reason of how much debate came to rest on this particular point, as Michael Mulkay usefully documents in his detailed monograph devoted to this issue (1997). For many, including Warnock herself, the prominence of the embryo question came as something of an unexpected development. (It was, in part, the question of why it did so which initially drew me to this debate as one I saw as being about an 'unfamiliar kinship'). Following the HFEA, use of the (British) distinction between embryos and 'pre-embryos', determined by the appearance of the primitive streak (the emergent spinal column visible at approximately two weeks' development) has become an internationally recognised standard for the governance of assisted reproduction.

The limit of fourteen days was, of course, one of many established within the Act. One way to describe the HFEA is as an elaborate set of delimitations. Limits were set to prohibit interspecies fertilisation, cloning and so forth – often with the aim of reassuring an anxious public. One of many limits established by Parliament was how long an embryo could be stored – a five-year limit was enacted on embryo storage.[2]

The limit on embryo storage reached its first horizon in August 1996 – five years from the inauguration of the Authority in August 1991. A minor modification of legislative procedure in 1996 entitled couples to file written consent to allow embryos to be stored for a further period of up to ten years or donated for research purposes. Otherwise, they would be 'allowed to perish'. This legal limit catapulted embryos into public debate once again, in August 1996, as the spectre of thousands of frozen embryos being removed from their cyropreserved slumber and discarded provided irresistible media headlines.[3] So-called 'orphan' embryos garnered substantial television, radio and newsprint coverage, fuelled by the drama of a countdown to locate thousands of couples, in Britain and elsewhere, whose written consent was required to prevent a thawing of would-be progeny described by the Pope as 'genocide'.

Again, it is outside the remit of a brief afterword to account for the complex dimensions of indecision, non-decision, hesitation or desperation visited upon the embryo custodians implicated in this event. Whether they were clinicians, embryologists, administrators or former IVF clientele, the occasion was clearly fraught with conflicting impulses. What is certain is that this enactment of limitations – the need to destroy stored embryos – now occurs annually, thus producing a classically overdetermined reproductive dilemma. It turns out that a necessary element in the governance of technologically assisted conception is a limit to population growth in the form of the annual disposal of stored embryos.

The perspective offered in the preceding chapter argues that the question of embryonic human existence is vexed because it is relational, and because the context of this relationality is unfamiliar. The question this volume as a whole addresses is not only how well individuals or families, institutions or governments, or Parliament and the medical or legal professions, adjudicate responsibility for technologies of procreation under novel conditions of choice, responsibility, accountability or efficiency. In the research conducted for this collaborative study, we used divergent contexts to investigate the terms through which such dilemmas are imagined and addressed.

It turns out that the questions raised by kinship in the context of NRTs cannot be understood in the narrow sense of how 'the technological', or technological 'assistance', has altered the terrain of reproductive choice. We needed instead to examine how technological innovation enacts and materialises particular kinds of cultural values, including what appeared to emerge publicly as deeply held convictions about the human condition, such as the unique value placed on scientific progress in the name of increasing human knowledge, the importance of the desire to reproduce, and the need for limits on the technological manipulation of human life. We have argued that the means through which such conflicting values become part of the procreation of new persons, whereby a new generation of persons is brought into being who embody these uncertainties, is a far more complex process of cultural change than can be encompassed by a problematic defined simply in terms of the discovery of new techniques of human fertilisation and the need to regulate them.

It now appears, five years after we originally published this study, that particular kinds of *cultural drift* not only affect, but are built into, the governance of human fertilisation and embryology. That is to say, limits seem to reproduce other limits: they have a life of their own. It is clearer now that it is not only a new population of persons born of assisted conception techniques who embody the cultural values of kin connection, the desire to reproduce, or the importance of scientific progress and technological innovation. These values also affect our relation to a somewhat unexpected population: a population of thousands of frozen embryos in indefinitely cryopreserved suspension.

The difficulties encountered in the context of discarding frozen embryos make explicit a paradoxical relationship between respect for human life and the capacity of technology to enable its creation. There is evident public concern that technologies of procreation be subject to governance. But the governance of life turns out to include an annual mandate for death. There is no reason to remove an embryo from storage other than a legal one, based on moral imperatives, such as the necessity of limits. Yet these limits derive from an intensity of respect for technologically created life as a means to relieve infertility and to alleviate the suffering caused by genetic pathology.

This too turns out to be an important source of cultural drift, for it is in the context of assisted conception that we see more clearly how culture is itself a technology – an implicit analogy that runs throughout our discussions. Like technology, culture is a source of innovation, and as in the context of technology, innovation is required. Culture in this sense is also 'like' procreation: it is a means of bringing forth. The ricochet, to use Marilyn Strathern's phrase, of these analogies is not a matter of merely academic interest. As this intra-contextual study demonstrates, a vast empirical dimension to this 'ricochet effect' is evident in the many forms through which people reflect upon and implement such connections and disconnections. Documenting this process shows us more than how technology *reflects* cultural values: it demonstrates *how the workings of culture can be made evident through its technologies,* and in this case also *how such transformations come to be embodied.*

Kinship in the context of NRTs is therefore wrongly understood merely to describe the immediate kinship-related dilemmas occasioning novel forms of assisting the conception of new persons, through techniques such as IVF.[4] The approach taken here raises a different set of questions about the forms of cultural knowledge mobilised in and around such practices. People who have no direct contact with techniques such as IVF are quick to recognise themselves to be affected by them none the less. In turn, these forms of recognition can be collected, described, analysed and pondered as episodes which bring elementary questions about late-twentieth-century cultural change into sharper focus.

One way to approach the question of how people make sense of new means of producing life and death is that they may know more than we think. One method to explore this possibility is to examine how kinship is used as a context for understanding. It turns out that kinship is alive and well in the age of assisted conception, much as the connections it is being used to trace are relatively unfamiliar. It turns out for the anthropologist that kinship is, among other things, both a system for determining connections, and as such a unique point of reference for making sense of a world far beyond the kinship universe of what is most familiar.

NOTES

1 A detailed account of the passage of the Human Fertilisation and Embryology Act is provided in Morgan and Lee (1991). See also Gunning and English (1993) for an account of the history of the regulation of in vitro fertilisation in Britain. For accounts of the debate specifically concerning embryo research, see Mulkay (1997) and Spallone (1996).
2 This limit on storage was initially suggested by the Warnock Committee for two reasons: because of the unknown consequences of freezing an embryo on

a subsequent offspring, and because of the legal complications potentially consequent upon separation or divorce of the couple by whom the embryo was created.

3 The precise number of 'orphaned' embryos 'allowed to perish' in August 1996 is the subject of on-going uncertainty. Estimates range from 3 to 12,000.

4 There is a rapidly expanding ethnographic literature on assisted conception. Studies such as those by Cussins (1996, 1998), Kahn (1997), Inhorn (1994, 1996), Inhorn and Van Balen (1999), Ragoné (1994), Sandelowski (1993), and my own account of IVF (1997) provide ethnographic analysis of the encounter with assisted conception at the point of consumption.

5 Regulation, substitution and possibility

Marilyn Strathern

> In this conception, each individual . . . is best thought of as a node in an overall hereditary web. Linking the nodes within the web there are kin relationships among members of a generation and also between succeeding generations.
>
> (Grobstein 1990: 20)

This could come from almost any account of Euro-American life. It echoes the description of kin networks of the kind familiar to anthropologists since Firth and his colleagues' (1969) classic exposition on family and kinship in London. It also echoes a recent reformulation made in the context of a historical sociology of family relationships in 'Western' societies (in this instance Britain and North America). Goldthorpe (1987: 4–5) observes that, as kinspersons, family members are linked not as a group but as a network. They constitute a set of people to whom 'an individual' ought to be able 'to turn for help and support' and expects to do so on a reciprocal basis. Unlike other forms of assistance, such support carries the long perspective of a lifetime, and this, he suggests, is 'the prime importance of kinship in Western [Euro-American] societies'.

However, Grobstein is neither anthropologist nor sociologist. Now in a Program in Science, Technology and Public Affairs in California, he was trained in embryology and developmental biology, and I have taken his remarks from an address to a British-based conference on philosophical ethics in reproductive medicine (Bromham *et al.* 1990). The individual to which he was referring is not a person but the 'individual genome' that every person carries. He thus visualises kinship as lying between the sets of hereditary material themselves (the genomes). Grobstein produced this image in the context of an appeal to what he hoped would be taken for granted in future debate, namely the idea that the human genome is a fundamental collective property that belongs to and links all humanity. He might, therefore, have been gratified to have heard some of the speakers in the House of Lords claim their connectedness through the identity they shared with the embryo under discussion.

Grobstein ends his address by suggesting the need for a regulatory body that could formulate a prospectus for the role and limits of intervention, as he puts it, in the human future. That might be essential, he adds, 'to proceeding with due caution to reap the benefits while avoiding the hazards of our dawning use of genetic intervention in our own fundamental continuity and kinship' (1990: 23). What he says about genetic manipulation has been echoed in other areas of reproductive medicine, including the fertility treatment services which have given us our examples in this book, and was echoed in the parliamentary discussion. What is interesting about his statement is the way in which an appeal to limits is couched in terms of an explicit reminder of humanity's 'kinship'.

Grobstein does so by drawing on two kinds of fact. On the one hand he describes an uncontroversial and taken-for-granted natural fact. The genome is there before the person; the links between the nodes of the hereditary web are there before human beings start thinking about them. Kinship in this sense is no hypothesis, and is not put forward as a representation of anything else: it simply refers to the biological ramifications of genetic inheritance. On the other hand, however, he wishes that the knowledge will be put to use in a certain way. Grobstein not only assumes that the links and webs have meaning, but regards them as imposing an obligation on people.[1] In becoming the foundation of an appeal, kinship as a biological fact is also rendered a social fact. More than that, it is on the basis of already existing kinship among all of us that he specifically appeals for help and support. If we realise we are all related, he implies, we should also realise our common cause.

This chapter comments on two phenomena already evident in these remarks; both are intrinsic to the place that kinship has in the formulation of possibilities in reproductive medicine. One is the recurrence of similar observations across diverse contexts, the 'echoes' that appear to connect them. The other is the differentiation that appears between kinds of facts, as between the 'natural' facts of linkage and the 'social' meanings put on them. Indeed, whether we are talking of contexts or facts, connection and differentiation proceed together.[2] This is especially true when one kind of knowledge is regarded as a foundation for another. My aim is to elucidate both.

Euro-American ideas about kinship rest on multiple orderings of knowledge. What enables Grobstein to give his special reading of hereditary links between genomes also informs understandings of kinship itself. In summoning 'kinship', people may be summoning the concrete relational world in which they live – the relatives they have to deal with, the dependants they care for, the obligations that follow expectations of support and help. But they also entertain ideas about the substantial links (including but not exclusively genetic ties) there are between kin (why the network is there in the first place), and can think of these in an abstract way as facts of life that affect everyone.[3] This abstract knowledge – exactly as Grobstein hoped would also be true of knowledge about our common ancestry – is not neutral. It has consequences for the way actions are judged. The fact that people are related puts them into a relationship that cannot be ignored. There is thus already a limit to what, as kinspersons, they can do.

How should we address the differences between knowledge? Debate over the new reproductive technology (NRT) is constituted in the way that diverse facts are introduced, and diversity does not simply lie in the difference between natural and social ones: there are differences between various natural facts that are held to ground social ones, as there are differences between the social relevance of the meanings put on them and the contexts in which they occur. In so far as we can identify particular purposes or motivations in the way people draw on one area rather than another, we may refer to different domains or orders of knowledge. (At a later point it will be useful to draw a distinction between domains and orders.) Limits do not exist simply as regulations on what people are prepared to do: they also exist in such domaining of knowledge. The materials offered in this book show certain strategies of domaining at work.[4] They also show how people move between orders of knowledge. Persons may be hoping to make everything relevant to what they want to say, or they may hope to narrow the relevance of what they wish to consider so as to contain its implications. The interplay between these possibilities is of particular significance to the understanding of how kinship is treated. For kinship is often understood as simultaneously ubiquitous in society and outside areas of principal public concern.[5]

Let me return to the aims of this chapter. In the course of elucidating these points, we shall find that what began as a solution also becomes a problem. The Introduction suggested that it is possible to make sense of people's concerns by putting them into context. As far as the eliciting of information is concerned, we have presented four diverse contexts. The materials reported on here were derived by quite different means from the clinicians and parliamentarians described in Chapters 1 and 4 from those whose views are presented in Chapters 2 and 3; and so forth. *Contextualisation renders each set intelligible.* At the same time, the explorations that characterised our approach to the data have also revealed the extent to which similar concerns flow across the four contexts.[6] And at this point, the solution offered by the earlier analysis of contextualisation becomes the problem. There are connections between these different contexts, though there is no supra-context to contain them all. If we think of ideas about NRT providing the common context, it is one that partially connects rather than encompasses the others.[7] What then becomes evident is that we are dealing with the way our subjects themselves contextualise their approach to this issue; if so, their exclusions work to render certain views 'invisible'. *Contextualisation prevents connections from being made.* In a field that affects us all, as Grobstein said, we cannot afford that.

Our hope is that the present exercise may throw light on some of the processes at work in public debate and in the application of different know-ledges. If solutions in one area turn out to be problems in another, this is as true of the developments in the NRTs themselves as it is of the way they become part of social and cultural life.

CONTEXTUALISATION: THE CONCERN WITH LIMITS

The Foreword to the Warnock Committee's Report (1985: 2) voices what is presumed to be a common concern:

> [I]t would be idle to pretend that there is not a wide diversity in moral feelings, whether these arise from religious, philosophical or humanist beliefs. What is common . . . is that people generally want *some principles or other* to govern the development and use of the new techniques. There must be *some* barriers that are not to be crossed, *some* limits fixed, beyond which people must not be allowed to go. Nor is such a wish for containment a mere whim or fancy. The very existence of morality depends on it. [Original emphasis.]

Yet limits do not exist in a vacuum any more (as the report goes on to point out; and see Dyson 1990) than morality does. They are created out of the constraints that people impose on themselves by the very nature of their sociality. To live a social life is to move between experiences that impinge on persons from diverse origins and to diverse effect. That diversity rests on a sense of the distinctive or intrinsic character of particular actions and values. Indeed, at the heart of the Warnock Inquiry and the legislation that ensued is the assumption that limits are not set by the technologies themselves but must come from other domains of social life.[8] So what character would the kinds of limits Warnock mentions have; how might they be articulated?

Regulation

At the end of one of Eric Hirsch's conversations, something was said that raised the possibility of an inadvertent joining of reproductive material which would have been incestuous. The inference about incest arose from the kinship identity of the persons involved. Uttering that inference acted as a spoken limit to what the couple whom Hirsch was interviewing were prepared to countenance. It would be morally unthinkable to facilitate such a union. Here we have an example of the feeling that there should be some limit 'beyond which people must not be allowed to go', and a concrete articulation of the way limits are set by prior kin relations.

It is a long-established supposition in the Euro-American cultural reper-toire that the institutions of kinship and family 'regulate' biological pro-cesses for social ends.[9] Regulation exists in the way relationships are defined and negotiated, and in the expectations attached to them. This no more so than when the manner of regulation is under dispute. Elliot (1986: 1) opens her account of change and continuity in 'the family' thus: '[I]n many modern Western societies, the *regulation* of sexual parental relationships has become the subject of vigorous and heated debate' (my emphasis). She is referring to a contrast between 'traditional' and 'alternative' family styles.

If kinship is thought to have a regulatory function in the strong sense, it also implies regulation in a weak sense. To introduce the topic of kin rela-tionships is at the same time to introduce a domain of life that has a char-acter of its own, and is thus governed by its own conventions. So when it is brought into view, then its own complex internal structure invites ramifica-tion. For example, as soon as one thinks about the possibility of relatedness existing without being known, then other unknowns come into the picture, such as the sexual secrets of private life. People in Alltown were ready with extrapolations. When they were thinking of the identity of the parties involved, gamete donation might cross the barrier into adultery, or conjure up inappropriate couplings between the generations or an unequal balance between in-laws. And the child that had the potential to create links (make relationships) could by the same token also be seen as disrupting links (already based on relatedness). In the context of thinking about kinship, one set of problematics thereby leads into another. This was eloquently articulated by Snowden (1990: 78) at the conference noted earlier. In spell-ing out the implications of semen donation for the donor's kin, he points to endless social ramifications – for the wife (who may be disturbed at the thought of unknown offspring), for his parents (who have unknown grand-children), for his own children (and their missing half-siblings), and so on. Consequences ramify as far as kin relationships ramify.

These relationships already exist and have their own character. It is a characteristic of the network formation of kin relations that they ramify (cf. C. Harris 1990: 62). It is the pre-existence of these relationships that sets limits to how new opportunities (such as egg donation) present themselves. Our studies describe some of the cultural attributes that both define the domain of kinship and connect it to other domains which make kinship a particular medium through which people might think about the need for regulation.

First, it is evident that we are dealing with hopes as well as fears, with perceived benefits as well as problems. Alltown people (Chapter 2) are specific on this point. Both the hopes *and* the fears are embedded in ideas about the relatedness of persons, and in the way in which persons locate themselves in unique constellations of kin. Inasmuch as the new fertility treatments offer people the chance to complete their families, or otherwise become a parent, then they remedy conditions that may arise in anyone from any class or background. For although it is recognised that people live out diverse family lives, the Euro-American convention would take a desire to reproduce as thoroughly natural. Hence the common conflation of infertility and childlessness (Franklin 1990: 219). Yet these two components of kinship thinking – having children to complete a family and the desire to reproduce – produce the diverging perspectives on the 'suitability' of persons for treatment voiced in Chapter 1. A necessity to impose some kind of limit appeals to the relational environment in which children will grow up, while questions about the appropriateness of any limit appeal to the individual's desire to be a parent. Reservations about money being the discriminatory factor in who will benefit are raised in Chapter 3.

This leads, second, into the question of desire itself. Several of the couples to whom Hirsch spoke raise questions about consumerism. An important component of the kinds of sentiments that flow between parents and children, at least in the English version of Euro-American kinship, turns on the ideal that children are wanted by their parents. Conversely, the 'mother' is constructed as having maternal impulses that are only fulfilled by having a child. Yet many people suggest that such thoroughly human desires may themselves need regulating; they should not be seen to be satisfied by any means possible. Thus it is thought to be inappropriate to express them in the same way as one might express a desire for commodities that (a typical example) the supermarket made available. Unlimited choice is seen as problematic. Here, then, the commercialisation of fertility treatment indicates not limits on availability but the limitless nature of availability when all that would act as a brake would be cash. As Gloria de Guy said, '[for many], it's like you get a car, a dishwasher and then a dog *and then you think what next*?' (p. 115, my emphasis).

Third is the traditional relationship between sex and reproduction. Here, prior relationships may exist either through ties of substance or the marriage contract. Socially inappropriate desires, or thought inappropriate by some, have always been signalled by the negative concepts of incest and adultery. In this world view, procreation is a sexual act, as well as a reproductive one, and Euro-American ideas about kinship are also ideas about sexual partnership. Edwards and Hirsch make it clear that in thinking through the relational consequences of certain procreative possibilities, people may position the parties involved as though donors and recipients of gametes were instead partners to a sexual act. What seems at issue is less the propriety of the partners' actions than the consequences for the combination of substances. For the topic of incest was frequently raised in the context of anonymity. The anonymity that protects donors and recipients from thinking about themselves as sexual partners at all, and thus protects the act of fertilisation from the intimacy of a social relationship, works because it is also assumed there is no prior genetic relationship between them. It obviously does not apply to persons who know they are already related. And anonymity itself becomes problematic when it conceals the knowledge by which one would determine in the future whether persons about to embark on a sexual partnership were genetically (already) related or not. Some of those with whom Edwards spoke in effect raised the question of having to think about relating to, and relationships between, not persons as such but gametes themselves (what 'name' they would carry) because of the consequences of inappropriate or unknown combinations. At the same time, the break between the act of conception and the birth of the child could lead to the anomalous situation of persons knowing there were others to whom they were linked through 'conception' rather than 'a birth' (p. 74).

Fourth, then, is the part that knowledge itself plays in Euro-American kinship. Alltown people are thoroughly sceptical about concealing knowledge in the long term. But there is also the worry that knowledge may come too late (and see p. 76). However, if people are troubled at the thought of anonymous semen donation leading to inadvertent situations where siblings unknowingly marry, it cannot be because of the likelihood of that happening. Everyone would agree it is remote. Rather, it must be because ideas about appropriate procreative partners are part of further ideas *about how you 'know'* who is or is not related. The way in which you know who is or is not a kinsperson, intrinsic to the definition of identity, traditionally introduces different kinds of facts. There is a difference between the presumed fact that everyone is born of two genetic parents and the way in which you prove the identity of this or that individual parent. Maternity traditionally is 'known' in different ways from paternity.[10] The mother is evident from having given birth, whereas the father is defined through his genetic contribution. Since the genetic contribution is ordinarily established through acts that remain private to the individual persons concerned, public acknowledgement of the father has to rest on knowledge about the relationship between partners.

Fifth, Alltown people brought home the whole question of ownership. The connections that lie between kin are conceptualised in terms of their 'belonging' to each other. As Edwards explains, such claims imply a mutual identification through relationship. Here knowledge about origins is critical for the way in which kin identify themselves with one another, as the Berkshire Doles (Chapter 3) also presume. Indeed some Alltown residents, such as Veronica Thomas, go so far as to suggest that people's individuality would be compromised by their not knowing exactly how they were made up. Despite the immediacy of her language, she is speaking here in highly abstract terms. Several discussions bring up other circumstances, such as adoption, where knowledge about ancestry is incomplete or withheld and – for all the issues it raises – does not compromise the person's sense of individuality. But these are taken as the accidents of life. A critical difference, mentioned in both Chapters 2 and 3, lies in the idea that persons might be procreated by strangers ('scientists') who had no interest in the social identity of the child. As a consequence, persons themselves would be unregulated, so to speak, by not knowing to whom they belonged.

And, sixth, the idea of kinship itself evokes links and ties which are already there – that is, have been laid down by previous generations. It is because of this that kinship looks backwards as well as forwards. Paula Seddon referred to a woman who acted as kin-keeper as someone who was 'a touch with the past' (p. 70). On-going family life might be 'a project' (p. 103), but it is one instigated by prior (genetic) connection. In turn, existing kinship links provide a kind of reservoir on which future links can draw. This can be imagined literally as a reservoir when egg donation between close relatives is being considered. The colloquialisms of a 'gene pool' (used by a clinician) or the family 'bloodline' (used by a client) are close to Grobstein's concept of a collective property. Genes are somehow thought of as bounded by their paths of transmission. Thus the bloodline may be conceptualised as descending from one's ancestors as though it were their identities that were being projected forward. The sense of priority that Alltown people referred to as 'roots' rests on the fact that kin links are those links already in place. That priority gives substance to the sense of limitations being set by existing relationships.

Although I have numbered these points, this is not a list that could ever be complete. What it shows are some of the ways in which kinship works as a context in which, through their management of relations with one another, people feel constrained by pre-existing limits. Limits are also recognised when people become conscious of crossing over into other (pre-existing) domains of life so that 'other' factors, such as distaste for consumerism or fear of strangers' intentions, are thought to challenge what kinship is supposed to be about. Yet to perceive such boundary crossing as limiting rather than liberating raises the question of conservatism.

When kinship becomes the background to other opportunities in life, it is an English convention to perceive relations to family and kin as holding the individual back, as brakes on innovation and independence, as links that are also, literally, ties.[11] The very term 'limit' conjures it all. Since this book focuses on present practice rather than future possibilities, and on English versions of Euro-American cultures rather than on a wider world stage, and especially since it focuses on kinship, the concept of conservatism is in need of clarification.

Conservatism and innovation

The absence of intrinsic limits to change was an issue on which many in the parliamentary debates spoke. Sarah Franklin quotes Sir Ian Lloyd's positive view: 'For us to forswear the assistance which science can provide in modifying that [genetic] code to the advantage of the human race would be an indefensible abdication of responsibility' (p. 147).

It is a powerful appeal to innovation to suggest that if we were not to seize present opportunity, we would be cheating future generations. As J. Harris (1992: 5) says of biotechnology, how the new powers that we can already anticipate will be used will depend in large part on political decisions, and those in turn on the power of arguments for and against their use. It would be conservative for the sake of it to make arguments turn on ideas about the conduct of human relationships simply because they are in place. '[W]ho's to say the barriers won't move?' (Maria Williams, p. 117). Precisely because they are already in existence, current concepts may thus seem a barrier in the way of progress or development. A time lag between the conditions of life to which people are accustomed and the possibilities opened up by the NRTs may, so it seems, be inevitable, but equally inevitably, so it seems, the gap will close. Denis White observed: 'We probably need time to catch up with the medical people . . . given enough time, we will all start to think differently' (p. 118).

Yet a cultural account can only address ideas that are already in place. This appears doubly true of kinship. The sixth feature of kinship thinking to which I drew attention is also part of a general set of associations that is certainly English if not more widely Euro-American. Kinship is to do with continuity, ancestry and tradition (this is what makes the family so apparently susceptible to breakdown in the face of innovation), and tradition is by turn comforting and stultifying. Such representations of the past and future have a long history. Novelty and newness substantively 'cover' this history with their connotations of a destabilised and innovative world of possibilities. Tradition goes the other way: however innovative people's use of it, the concept evokes and is thus intended to 'reveal' past practice.[12] It would therefore seem that the topic of kinship is bound to belong to a world already passing. By comparison, the idea of the future itself underlines the potential reach of human possibility. Future possibilities make current practices seem at once parochial and limited.

Against such a background, *the NRTs themselves provide a new context* in which to think about human affairs. In so far as the NRTs enable Euro-Americans to do things they could never have done before, they bring new sets of assumptions into place, and in doing so create the sense of conservatism that is attached to the old. In this view, novel possibilities are opened up for realising people's desires.[13] In so far as the NRT's intervene in the processes of procreation, then, they do not simply validate old representations of what kinship is about. They have the potential to make us think again about what we take for granted, what we look for in family life, how we regard the relationship between parents and children. In short, they offer a context that will give its own shape to the way Euro-Americans think about kin.

This sense of possibility is evident in the material that Franklin examined. The NRTs provide a new context for thinking about human reproduction; but what kind of context is it? Franklin argues that it is a context with a special characteristic. It offers the possibility of *lifting* what used to be limits on what persons could do. The limits are, in the first place, natural/ biological ones; in the second place they are the old limits on the way people reacted to the coming into being of family life. One piece of knowledge that the NRTs bring, then, is that there need be nothing constant in the relationship between natural facts and the social relations built on them.[14] So when they serve as a context for thinking about other things, the NRTs present the paradox of a context whose rationale of boundless opportunity is substantively 'about' decontextualisation.

Like any new context, this one works in so far as it is not contained by other contexts but rather gathers to itself information, values and ideas from many, and thus appears to deal with elements from each of them in a decontextualised way. But, in addition, it would seem that its essence is to hold out possibilities for action that are unbounded. Attached to the idea of development in this field is the very potential for breaking bounds – hence the fantasy of human 'cloning'. (Cloning is raised by people both as an indication that there are no intrinsic limits to what is possible, and as a scare word that everyone will recognise as indicating the need for some outer limit.) As I noted earlier, it has to be domains recognisable from other areas of social life that are brought to bear, so that their reference to other values constitutes a limit to what otherwise seems open to endless extension. (In the cloning example, it is values attached to individual diversity.) Such domains include the parliamentary decision-making process itself: 'The Bill gives us a firm foothold. It gives the public and the scientist the certainty that they want' (p. 148).

I shall return to the question of decontextualisation. First, I wish to comment on the equation between the unbounded and the innovatory, and the part that existing cultural concepts play in the imagining of future possibilities. Hirsch reminds us of constructions of modernity. Modernity supposes a divide between the 'traditional' and the 'modern'. Yet moderns imagine they can destabilise the claims of the past in the present when in doing so they are destabilising their claims to innovation: as Franklin makes evident, reproductive medicine requires those very ideas that it upturns. What emerged from our studies more generally is the extent to which kinship, far from being put on one side, is made relevant to the kind of future certain people imagine for themselves. They are not alone in this.

J. Harris provokes his readers to think the unthinkable, to release themselves from previous habits of thought, by a new and apparently unbounded idea:

> [B]irth has operated as a traditional divide. In law it marks the distinction between the offences of abortion and infanticide and most people celebrate birth as the arrival of the new human individual. We may be on the verge of an era in which ectogenesis, the nurturing to term of the fetus in an artificial womb, will be possible. When this happens the notion of birth will lose much of its legal and social significance.
>
> (1992: 1)

One practice (birth) loses its social significance while another (ectogenesis) acquires it. Harris's intention was to underline the extent to which current moral categories are, as he puts it, in disarray. Yet it would seem that the notion of 'birth' can only be destabilised ('lose much of its legal and social significance') if legal and social significance continue to be given to 'nurturing', 'the fetus' and 'womb'.[15] Ectogenesis then becomes a substitute for birth.

To give new forms significance through old ones is to mobilise already existing cultural suppositions. To ask of a fertilised egg in a petri dish whether it is a person is to ask a question one might in the past have asked of a fetus quickening in the womb. Or to assume that embryo implantation raises questions about whether or not the implantee is the mother is to draw the act into the realm of family relationships (cf. Wolfram 1987: 212). And the particular kind of connection being made between old and new forms of expression is likely to be especially relevant to procedures of evaluation or assessment. Thus Haimes (1990: 155) discusses 'the way reproductive technologies, though "new" in their technical aspects, are assessed with reference to established notions about the norms of family life' (and see Cannell 1990). Her evidence comes from clinical, medical and policy discussions. There is still a connection even when the applicability of those norms is questioned, as it is by some of the clinicians with whom Price spoke: 'I feel very loath to apply rules [about the suitability of persons as parents] to the infertile when the fertile don't have these rules applied to them' (p. 37). The 'rules' are, of course, people's reference points, their means of representation and thus their already existing suppositions. Along with such suppositions invariably comes more than seems asked for. Clinicians are aware of this in impressing the complications of IVF procedures on to the client who asks them simply to 'maximise my chances of getting pregnant' (p. 42).

Beyond the clinic, perhaps the mobilisation of new forms through old contributes to the sense of exaggeration with which people may emphasise that everything in this area is new – or else that nothing is. One may either distance the present from the past or regard current practice as continuous with it. Questions seem both new and old at the same time (Abrahams 1990).

It is frequently remarked that 'the NRTs' include old practices such as donor insemination. DI does not depend on technology the way that the use of eggs does, yet insemination in the context of the NRTs is caught up by the comparison, and may be regarded as part of medical procedure. Current regulatory arrangements, for instance, mean that as far as the medical profession is concerned, it can only be offered on licensed premises. One connection leads to another. The donation of semen may in turn offer a model for regarding egg transfer as 'donation' (but see Haimes 1991). Similarly, the fact that a person is 'assisted' to have a child can lead to the idea that nature itself is assisted, even though often the defective natural processes are bypassed and what is assisted is the wish to have a child (Morgan 1989: 59 refers to a previous 'procreative intent', and see the comments from Winston quoted on p. 37). 'Donation' and 'assistance' are terms familiar from human interactions: there is nothing new in either of them. It is, of course, their contextualisation that makes the difference.

When the basic ideas themselves seem old, then the emergent property of new procedures becomes that of capability. In extending capability, putting the realisation of desire in reach, the new technologies seem to offer solutions to perennial human problems. But this means that they are also shaped by old ways of conceptualising the human problems themselves (Stolcke 1986). For example, the fact that gamete transfer involving a third party is classified as a 'donation' also classifies it (in Euro-American terms) as the act of someone disposing of something that is alienable; this in turn raises the question of when it becomes a commodity rather than a gift, connecting it to a domain of values to do with the ethics of commercialisation. Classifications introduce their own connections.

Such connections are context-creating. We have seen that kinship evokes the idea of ideas already in place – what can be taken for granted – and thus a conservative area of possibilities. Traditional and customary ways are those thought to have been in place for a long time, that belong to convention and become outmoded by changing circumstances. Ideas seem old, then, precisely because they belong to an established context, and one that is recognisable as a context: a relatively bounded domain. We have also seen that the NRTs do not appear to work as such a 'context' in the same way. Rather, they appear as a range of possibilities that open up new vistas, and their open-endedness would make them the very reverse of a domain in this sense. Hence the Brave New World hopes about possibilities are also Hitleristic fears about where it will all lead, as observations made to Hirsch make evident. Yet the talk about hopes and fears for the future thereby mobilise images that have become almost culturally orthodox with respect to the NRTs. A similar cultural conservatism underlies the way the technologies themselves are argued about.

Anthropologists raise the question of cultural conservatism because they are interested both in the limits (culture) that people set on their lives and in how they enable themselves to live them (their conservation of themselves). So while on the face of it cross-cultural analysis would appear to open up radical and otherwise unthought possibilities, in fact this is simply the effect of anthropologists' interest in other people's cultural conservatism seen from the perspective of their own. In focusing on the conventions of Euro-American kinship, any anthropologist with cross-cultural and thus comparative expertise would acknowledge the former's specific and local character. Rivière, commenting among other things on possibilities in the conception of motherhood, puts the case for comparison succinctly:

> I am not advocating . . . that we should therefore adopt the ideas and practices of other people. I am merely suggesting that it might help if we removed our cultural blinkers and saw our problems in a wider perspective. If we did this, then surrogate mothers might not appear to be the threat to civilization that some people make them out to be.
>
> (1985: 6)

Cross-cultural knowledge of itself does not invite us to follow the paths of other cultures. Anthropologists do not imagine there is anywhere a rainbow world that existed *as* myriad possibility or that showed up nothing but the malleability of human design. As Rivière implied, to search for one would simply yield the limitations under which other people construe their existence: one would simply be borrowing other people's limitations.[16] Rather, it is important to acknowledge the conservative force of all ideas. People articulate ideas that address a world already imagined. The 'newer', or even the more outrageous, ideas are supposed to be, the more one can be certain that they only acquire that effect by working off old assumptions.

The acceptability of new reproductive technology is among other things based on the possibility of changing the world, as Sir Ian Lloyd hoped, for the better: to assist conception, to find out more about embryo development, to create persons healthy in new and unprecedented ways. What is being conserved in these desires are old assumptions[17] about human life, the future, the nature of personal identity and the virtues of knowledge.

Everything is new and nothing is new. The paradox posed by the 'implications' of the NRTs dissolves if one realises that conservation is itself a force for change. By constantly attempting to make sense of their circumstances, justify their actions, find reasons for their values, Euro-Americans conserve their sense of themselves in creating new contexts out of old ones. As Edwards observes, 'they model new possibilities on old facts' (p. 64). Already-existing understandings are thus extended and modified, and new possibilities take the place of – substitute for – old ones. The NRTs have invited a series of such substitutions, and I have argued that in so far as they comprise a perspective through which people comment on other things, we may treat 'the NRT' as a context of sorts. Where the Introduction suggested the extent to which the domain of kinship works as an analytical context for making intelligible people's diverse reactions towards reproductive technology, this chapter also suggests the extent to which the NRTs serve as a context for how people may think about kinship. As we have seen, it is a 'domain' of unbounded and unprecedented possibility. It invites people to link existing ideas in novel ways, but not to any single effect.

I have used the term domain[18] to indicate the manner in which sets of practices and expertise offer relatively discrete or self-contained ways of contextualising experience. Putting ideas or statements 'into their context' is a mode of rendering them intelligible by seeing how they 'fit' with other ideas or statements. However, persons move between contexts, and every individual person deploys multiple perspectives. Hence the possibility of contest (e.g. Hartouni 1991). Indeed, in a plural society, as Mary Dobbs observed, 'one has to look at things from other people's point of view' (p. 111). In so far as individual persons are regarded as a composite of different experiences and relationships (as Alltown residents expressed it), we may say they conserve their sense of themselves by the way they make connections across such domains. Domains are in this regard all available for connection and thus comparable to one another.

While the pluralism of perspectives could be attributed to the different social positions – different by gender, family experience, class and so forth – that persons occupy, we have wished to emphasise a separate dimension. *The NRT debates themselves create positions.* They render explicit cultural issues (such as the connection between social and natural facts) that invite address in their own diverse and contested manner.

The present study attempts to make the effects of this explicitness apparent. Each chapter has its own relatively self-contained purpose, relating to the way in which data were elicited. Each has also been at some pains to stress internal diversity, the difference between the views people express, and the different views any one individual person might express. The connections between the chapters therefore require comment. There are evident continuities of idiom or modes of expression – for example, in the way people use 'cloning' to hint at an excess of choice and control on the part of the authorities that deprives persons of the basis of their individuality. Authorities in control, the value of individuality, the spectre of cloning: Euro-Americans create new contexts for their understandings by the domains they connect together. We can talk of a cross-over or borrowing between domains.[19] The connections between these chapters thus invite the reader to read them culturally, that is, as though they (the chapters) were 'borrowings' from one another. The following section turns to the way in which the people whose views the chapters draw on make just such borrowings themselves through the models, comparisons and analogies they offer.

But borrowings do not simply extend understandings. They also work to substitutive effect. To bring together or connect things from different domains requires decontextualising an original usage, taking an item out of its 'original' place and putting it elsewhere. In appearing from 'elsewhere', it substitutes for what was otherwise in place.

Legislation affords an obvious example. Medical, legal and ethical considerations applied to the question of embryo research offer a conjunction of expertise recontextualised for the purposes of parliamentary debate. The resultant parliamentary expertise thus includes appeals to facts derived from diverse sources. These substitute for common-sense (and other) understandings already in place. So what constitutes the single domain of parliamentary debate are also the competing and combining expertises of theologians, embryologists, genealogists from the General Register Office and so forth. For their part, in contributing to common debate, each expert necessarily decontextualises his or her knowledge from its original context in order for it to find a place in the new. Knowledge is simultaneously recontextualised and decontextualised.

If recontextualisation is also decontextualisation, any one context thereby closes off others. This is why the contextualisation that appears as a solution to the interpretation of materials (making diversity intelligible) can also become a problem (it obscures the connections). However, as is true of those whose views are described in this book, people may seek such closure. One common form of closure is to impose limits on what is to be counted as relevant.

Far from wishing to bring everything into view, or make relations between all parts of one's life and experiences, one may feel circumscribed or bound by expertise or other circumstances to limit what one says. Views and ideas become prioritised: some seem more relevant than others, to come with more weight or truth, to be closer to experience, and so forth. While other domains may be acknowledged, they will be kept to the margins, seen as irrelevant to the concern in hand, regarded as lying outside one's competence. Here domains cease to be comparable. On the contrary, an incommensurability appears in the different things a person knows or is prepared to act on, and we may speak instead of *orders* of knowledge.

DECONTEXTUALISATION: MAKING AND UNMAKING CONNECTIONS

Let me give a brief instance of facts being brought together from different domains of knowledge to create a specific context, and how the same process from another point of view could be read as an inadmissible combination of elements from different orders. I refer to a dialogue, but not one we recorded. It comes from the same conference at which Grobstein spoke of the individual genome.

The following interchange took place between a British professor of Moral Theology and a member of the Norwegian Medical Research Council:

MAHONEY: [The embryo is] a human entity. It is human genetically. It is not yet individualised in the sense of irreversibly taking a shape beyond reduplication. Therefore, it is at some identifiable stage, before which, one can say of it, it is not yet a human individual . . .

SOLBAKK: In your definition of human being as an entity your argument is from a biological perspective. When you are speaking about a human being as an individual, you are using the metaphysical or ontological way of argumentation. I think you could be trapped in the argument as this kind of distinction is very problematic from a logical point of view.

MAHONEY: If this is confusion between a biological description and an ontological interpretation, the ontological interpretation of the idea of the individual requires a biological component, because we are talking not about angels but about humans. The Warnock Report itself . . . talks about the primitive streak and the fourteenth day as the beginning of individuation. Now that term is used biologically, therefore I think the ambiguity that you raise does not actually hold.

(Bromham *et al.* 1990: 98, 103–4)

Each speaker attempts to reduce ambiguity by substituting for the other's his own definition of the individuality at stake. But whereas Mahoney crosses contexts and regards the connection between different facts as intrinsic to the entity under discussion (the ontological definition requires a biological component), Solbakk strives to keep contexts apart (do not confuse biology and ontology). The one produces a combination of comparable domains; the other separates knowledge into different orders. The one thus connects contexts that the other would keep distinct.

The strategies through which people thereby make concrete their understandings has a parallel in metaphor or analogy. These are ways of making comparisons. They simultaneously create connections (suppose a similarity between elements) and recreate difference (the similarity only works because the domains retain their distinctiveness). It is when both processes are perceived at once that people are aware they are drawing an analogy or turn an image into a metaphor.[20] Thus it is possible to borrow metaphors or make analogies between what are otherwise seen as the distinct domains of social and biological facts; the possibility can be contested when these are presented instead as incommensurate orders of knowledge. As such, they command different expertise, and expertise in one may well preclude expertise in the other. Or expertise may be suspended: we can say that everyone is a kinship expert, but kinship is not always relevant to the task in hand.

Borrowing (between domains) and the process of inclusion and exclusion (between orders of knowledge) engage two modes of decontextualisation. While the first creates connections between different areas of social and cultural life, the second discourages people from making them.

Borrowing

Prompted by questions that Alltown residents had posed for her, Jeanette Edwards found herself in a conversation about gametes passing between kin (Chapter 2). Patrick Croft immediately compared the consequences with what had happened to him. His mother had only been a girl when she became pregnant, and he had been brought up by his grandmother. This provides Edwards with an example of how, when thinking about possibilities presented through technological developments in reproduction, people make analogies with what they already know. Issues to do with NRT are represented through a comparison with what are perceived to be the kind of problems raised in complex family types formed through (in this case) adoption.

This is also an instance of the manner in which abstract ideas are translated into the concrete circumstances of life. People bring their own experiences to bear on the issue; in effect they borrow from what already exists for them as knowledge. What already exists serves as a 'model'; that is, a source of description or representation. It gives Mr Croft the realisation that 'in a way' that was 'exactly' what happened to him (p. 70). Thus does he draw an analogy between gamete donation among kin and the kinds of adjustments his mother and grandmother made at his own birth in order to press home a point about the categorisation of relatives. (One of the consequences he felt was that he has no 'full' brothers and sisters.) A model for such modelling lies in the way in which people compare different kinds of kin, such as step-kin or in-laws who are treated 'as if' they were 'real' kin.

Analogies thus extend the field across which consequences of certain actions can be imagined. In drawing on their own experiences, the Doles (see Chapter 3) offered adoption as a solution to the problem of single persons wishing to be parents (the so-called 'virgin birth' mothers), and as the acceptable side of surrogate arrangements. However, they thought that adoption should really be an alternative to fertility treatment services. So their comparison works in a double sense. It brings to mind children similar to some of those created through assisted conception who are not ('fully') related to their parents as well as 'orphan' children who are in need of parents. At the same time, adoption is presented as a practical measure that would serve as an appropriate solution to childlessness. It is brought up to suggest what could stand in the stead of fertility treatment services. Here the model of adoption works to substitutive effect: it introduces another way of thinking about aspects of the NRT that would render the NRT unnecessary.

The same comparison or analogy, then, that 'extends' people's understandings of a particular practice by drawing in other domains of experience may thus also have a displacement effect, and offer a 'substitute' for previous ways of thinking. Let us see further how this works.

Comparisons or analogies may be introduced in the most fleeting manner – a brief reference that summons other knowledge – but they may also evoke whole different worlds and their consequences. Already existing scenarios, in Hirsch's phrase, fuel the imagination. Scenarios are rather more than models, for they conjure up a set of circumstances that has its own internal narrative. They are also likely to serve as rather less than models, for they may summon circumstances of a notional kind (the ideal family) or of a kind that goes beyond experience (Brave New World). When Alltown residents compare 'scientists' to 'Hitler', they are invoking a historical figure who tried to alter the composition of an entire population; but the comparison works as part of a cultural repertoire that uses 'Hitler' as a sign for power out of control, and may as well conjure not historical incidents but futuristic fears of what scientists might do with the power they already have. We can call these scenarios in so far as they exist in already narrated form. In this vein, pre-existing attitudes towards consumer society exist as an already rehearsed scenario, and one more likely to be attributed to other people's experiences than to one's own (as in the comments on tele-shopping, p. 94).

When people go outside their own experiences, then, analogies summon different worlds, other ways of thinking about things. Different worlds can be found in ideals, in projected futures or recollected pasts, or in descriptions of contemporary circumstances that apply to other people rather than oneself. The baseline for comparison is what one is used to. It is clear that people may envisage new possibilities as displacing present habits.

While they may be imagined as cataclysmic, displacements may also turn on small, apparently trivial innovations. Thus they may consist of little more than images being borrowed from other domains of life and introduced into unexpected contexts: one suggestion was that a hospital might go in for special offers in types of children. The fantasy consists in combining two very mundane images – hospitals facilitate birth and supermarkets put on special offers. One is invited to think that, in so far as both provide services for customers, special offers in a hospital would be no more out of place than people shopping around to find what suited their reproductive preferences. So a combination that is outside anyone's experience is created by bringing together two experiences of a very ordinary kind. But the example of baby shopping (and it cropped up over and again) was meant to shock. When the commercial idiom substitutes for other ways of expressing preference or exercising reproductive choice, it deliberately provokes a boundary-crossing between the domains of kinship and commerce that are ordinarily kept separate.

Similar comparisons are evident in the way some of the people encountered in the four studies contemplate gamete donation. When they speak favourably of donation between close relatives in order to keep the bloodline within the family, it seems a small step for a child to be born (say) from the eggs of one sister rather than another. But what is true for egg donation may be accentuated by comparison with semen donation; it would not be as straightforward between brothers – competitiveness between men is held to make this a bigger step. Where the identity or origin of gametes is deliberately screened off, and the gametes thus depersonalised, then substitution may be justified on the grounds of physical attributes. In clinical contexts, one donation may seem as good as another, or one type of sperm preferred over another on grounds of likely success at fertilisation. In the case of egg donation between sisters, however, it is precisely their identity that is crucial. Common genetic ancestry provides the context in which sisters appears substitutable, and makes it a small matter for the eggs of one to stand in the stead of the eggs of another. Yet that idea itself also shocks. For when they are thought of as individual persons, with their own lives, their own constellation of relationships, their unique circumstances, then persons should be treated as quite distinct from each other. It is regarded as a confusion to relate to *a person* as simultaneously an aunt and a sister.

We could introduce a comparison of our own, and say that in this respect an individual person is like a domain, a self-contained constellation of characteristics.[21] Hence the 'substitution' of one known person by another is like an inappropriate borrowing between domains that should be kept separate. Similarly, the reversal of inter-generational expectation in the case of mother–daughter assistance, and the incestuous connotation of parents and children as sexual partners, arises because – as individual persons – such relatives are already embedded in a context of particular relationships. Chapter 2 shows how those relationships may be said to give persons not just connections with others (which then appear compromised) but their own uniqueness. Conversely, anonymity depersonalises, that is, takes away from the individual person a unique source of identity.

Substitutions between either known kin or else unknown donors and recipients appear problematic when they (kin or donors and recipients) are recontextualised as individual persons. Uniqueness comes from a combination of the individual's own biography and his or her placement in a nexus of relationships. Yet the image of the individual produces its own substitutive effect. Let me finally point to a context where the very idea of the unique individual has displaced, and made other, some of these aspects of personhood.

The centrality of the embryo to the parliamentary debates (see Chapter 4) seems to have been carried by more than the fact that the Bill was focused on the consequences of embryo research. The embryo became a vehicle through which several issues about science, the future and the intercon- nectedness of humanity were discussed. As a symbol of shared humanity, its treatment was thought to reflect the morality society would want to extend to a whole range of persons (see pp. 142–3). The future of humanity imagined as the future of the embryo who would develop into a person, and research on the embryo thought of as a future – for good or ill – for scientific knowledge, thereby set up comparisons that brought disparate domains into conjunction. Franklin further wonders if part of the impetus of the parliamentary discussion did not derive from the persuasiveness of certain substitutions. She suggests that the embryo that stood as a meta- phor for all of humanity, or for the future of (scientific) knowledge, also presented a being at an early stage of development whose potential to become a person rendered it a kind of substitute for already-existing per- sons. 'We are, after all, the subsequent development of embryos,' said Audrey Wise (p. 150).[22]

Yet what is most apparent about the embryo conceptualised thus is a decontextualisation that makes it least like a person (cf. Dyson 1990: 99). It is not yet in the world of social relationships, and can be contemplated as an otherwise solitary individual. The 'mother' was brought into the debate as a reminder of the fact that the embryo was literally embedded in another person. Yet that same containment by the mother also contributes to its decontextualisation from a wider world of relationships, including with its mother, into which it will be born.[23]

The connection between personhood and individuality was stressed over and over again. However, in the case of the embryo, the importance of the individual's uniqueness could not be established as it was in other accounts (and came over most prominently in Chapter 2) through its placement in a network of (kin) persons. The uniqueness of the embryo had to be estab- lished by other means available in the cultural repertoire, and what was emphasised in this context was its biogenetic identity. Whatever side the debaters took, it was understood that this was already in place from such moment as the individuality of the discrete being could also be identified, whether in the 'genetic blueprint' or in its cellular manifestation. In other words, this self-contained individualism, like the embryo's apparently self- contained potential for development, was interpreted as a biological fact. To perceive its individuality in this sense was effectively to displace a relational view. In the stead of 'significant others' that some Members of Parliament brought into the picture, for others there was in Franklin's words 'nothing to point to but the embryo itself' (p. 155).

I have deliberately run together various contexts in which one might think about displacement as a particular effect of borrowing. They range from the literal substitutions of gamete material to the metaphorical substitution of ideas by ideas. But that is the way in which models, comparisons, analogies and scenarios inform understandings of new processes. The extent to which such borrowings are admissible or inadmissible is, of course, part of the negotiation of different kinds of knowledge. In borrowing what seems an apt analogy or making what seem inadmissible extrapolations by references to circumstances which could never exist, persons decontextualise and thus recontextualise the information they have. This is a conserving exercise in so far as new entities or ways of thinking are built up through combinations of already existing ones. Thus the values associated with providing parentless children with a proper family life are conserved in the rationalisation that they could be offered surrogacy arrangements. Boundaries between domains of experience (such as kinship and commerce) may be crossed (shopping and giving birth mutually recontextualise each other) or be drawn again (the difference between these domains is sustained). As in the instance of the individuality of the embryo, conservation may also take the form of marginalising one kind of information (a field of relationships) with respect to another (biogenetic identity). This ordering is the topic of the section that follows.

Inclusions and exclusions

In an interview with Frances Price, one IVF clinician voiced his reluctance to judge between people's intentions (see p. 37). He conveys the sense of working from incomplete information – echoing Wynne's observation about how incomplete knowledge is pressed into policy use. Here it was a case of making decisions as to who should receive fertility treatment. The problems that counsellors talk through with intending clients are also problems that the clinician may discuss with counsellors. One expert, the clinician, thus draws on another, the counsellor, for advice. Judging the personal circumstances which make people seek fertility treatment was clearly felt to lie outside this clinician's competence: they belonged to another domain. As he observed, how to deploy this other information then becomes problematic. What information should be used to 'exclude' people from treatment? The necessity for priority entails an ordering of knowledge.

Beyond the need for statutory recognition (Price 1988: 38), slow as this has been (cf. Yoxen 1990), a more general 'need for regulation' is sometimes expressed by those working in IVF clinics. In Chapter 1, Price relates this to the extent that interpretation of good practice was, and continues to be, largely in practitioners' hands. While guidelines now govern the handling of embryos, the concern which clinicians continue to voice is their own understanding of how the decision to have a child is embedded in other domains of life. As a result, what is thoroughly contextualised by the clinic in terms of the drive to remedy infertility becomes problematic when it is recontextualised in terms of the chances of (say) multiple pregnancy and the life the multiparous parents will lead. Indeed, the desire to become pregnant may appear decontextualised from the desire to have a family in the understood sense.[24] In any event, clinicians raise what for them is the problematic issue of how to interpret the stated wishes of parents-to-be. What appears as a preference at one stage (the desire to become pregnant outweighing all other considerations) may look very different at other stages (when people think in the abstract about having triplets, for instance, or when they take triplets home). There will be cases, then, when the clinicians' problem is that they are dealing with clients who decontextualise their need to have children from other domains of life, including everything else that is associated with family and kinship relations. Perhaps some of the dilemmas on which Price reports are to do with the appropriateness of their wondering what context to put such desires into.

However sensitive they are to such issues, IVF practitioners may find themselves involved in their own decontextualisations. They may be aware of having to take decisions over the inclusion and exclusion of information; but they may also draw on orderings of knowledge that they take for granted. Thus the IVF clinician whose reluctance to judge has already been noted was at the same time giving priority to one interpretation at the expense of another. The client was said to want a child 'for herself', and for reasons of companionship – that otherwise she would be lonely in her old age. An anthropologist might interpret this as a desire for a relationship. At least as he reports it himself, the clinician understood the woman's desire as 'intensely self-centred' and by implication selfish (p. 38). This echoes the theme of the diverse scenarios on which Hirsch reports: the relative visibility of the individual as opposed to society. In this ordering, only the individual is 'seen': what is excluded is the social dimension to relationships themselves.

We do not, of course, have the rest of the evidence that either clinician or counsellor did in this case. But there is nothing in the words used to describe the woman's attitude that could not be accommodated within kinship idioms we have already come across. Quite apart from the point that kin are characterised as having obligations towards one another of a diffuse and enduring nature, which makes the woman's expectation of care in her old age culturally recognisable, the idea of persons 'belonging' to one another expresses the kind of appropriate attachment that makes the difference between real individuals embedded in a network of relations and free-floating, unattached entities. As we have seen, Alltown people convinced Edwards that a significant mark of individuality itself was the very centredness of persons that locates them in relation to others. And as one woman remarked to Hirsch: children are separate individuals 'but they are still part of you' (p. 107).

Yet if such kinship ideas seem excluded from the clinician's interpretation, perhaps it is for the very reason that Hirsch's study tries to make explicit: it may not be apparent that persons are speaking with other persons in mind, just as when looking at an individual one may not think of their being connected to others. The reason lies in a very general ordering of knowledge. From the way they talk, Euro-Americans often interpret one another's presence in a literal-minded sense and, as a consequence, may not 'see' the other persons or the connections unless an individual appears to be explicitly behaving in an other-directed manner. Yet it is clear from at least some of our fellow Euro-Americans, among those whose views are reported here, that references *to the individual person can imply a relational field* whether or not the field is specified. The exclusions that derive from ordering knowledge in such a way as to prioritise 'the individual', whose desire for a child comes to seem self-centred, are possibilities present in kin constructs themselves.

It would be a mistake to regard this particular prioritisation as a question of 'individualism' working *against* kinship. On the contrary, we have to see it as part of Euro-American kin constructs. As we have had cause to do elsewhere, we again draw on Schneider (1968) for his insights. Persons are relatives by certain kin criteria; but in this system relatives are also conceptualised as persons.[25] What Schneider epitomised for American kinship, Firth and his colleagues also established in their study of family and relatives in London. Speaking of the use of kin terms, they say this:

> What stands out in this English system is the tendency all the way through to specify persons individually, not give them a category term. Many societies seem to categorize kin and even to assimilate non-kin as quickly as possible into the kin-category scheme. They rarely use personal names even to children. All old men are 'grandfather'; all middle-aged men are 'father' or 'uncle' or 'father-in-law' . . . and so on. The middle-class English system can only do this in an informal context. In any formal context relatives must be properly pinpointed as individuals, with category label carefully qualified to bring out the personal aspect. In this sense the English kinship system can be called a *specifying system* as against the *categorizing systems* of many other, especially non-industrial, societies. But its specification is of individual persons, not statuses and roles.
>
> (Firth *et al.* 1969: 451; original emphasis)

This individualisation is replicated in myriad ways in which relatives deal with one another, such as the emphasis put on choosing whom to 'keep up with' or the emphasis on having a child that is one's own. Indeed, people's appreciation of the diversity of views and standpoints that others hold, the circumstances they find themselves in, the plurality of perspectives to which Edwards refers, is attributed to the individuality of persons: as she says, all kinds of social criteria are summarised as 'depending on the person' (p. 81).

This brings us to a crucial point. *The person can be thought of both as an individual entity and as an entity enmeshed in social relationships.* And this character of the Euro-American person is reproduced through kinship. Kinship – the way people think about and behave towards their families and relatives – is not the only place where such an entity is reproduced; but with its dual emphasis on the uniqueness of persons and their placement in a field of relations, kinship discloses both elements together.

Although he addresses himself to kinship in general, C. Harris's recent reconceptualisation of the topic has a particular bearing on how we might understand such Euro-American kin constructs. He would disagree with our characterisation of kinship as a 'domain' precisely on the grounds that it deals with relationships which are personal and therefore diffuse:

> All relationships which are 'personal' necessarily have a diffuse significance, since if the person, not the status, carries significance, then that significance cannot be confined to a specific social domain.
>
> (1990: 57)

What may not exist as a social domain may, of course, exist as a cultural domain among other cultural domains of knowledge, for reference may or may not be made to it. The issue will then be when and in what context 'personal' factors become relevant. The point that should hold our interest, however, is his characterisation of kinship relations as such. 'Kinship relations are *personal* relations, i.e. relations between total persons' (1990: 57; original emphasis). He adds that there is no context in which one could discount the fact of a relationship if it existed, any more than the relationship is ever the sole criterion on which a person acts.[26] In kin relations, then, orientation is towards the person, rather that towards the status or the act. He argues that this is what makes such relations unique. We would argue that it is also what makes the kin person unique: for the individual exists in a specific field of relationships that is already there.

If we here endorse the findings of earlier and other anthropological studies, then we do so to particular effect. It enables us to see the way in which some of the implications of the NRTs are rendered simultaneously socially visible and socially invisible. I return to the obvious fact that thinking of the person as both an individual and as engaged in social relations is not confined to kinship. Rather, this is a point of its connection with other domains of knowledge. Indeed, kinship is an exemplar of how *certain kinds of knowledge* are represented in this English version of Euro-American culture. When we look at the evidence that people draw on in thinking about the NRT, we find that *either social or individual factors may be classed as 'personal'*.

Such a convergence leads to interesting exclusions. It may be, as in the case mentioned earlier, that the reference to the 'self' (the woman's own desires) is taken as a reference to herself as an individual entity rather than as an (individual) person in a field of relationships. Here, the personal obscures the interpersonal. Or else, as the genre of personal opinions discussed in the Introduction attests, the way in which social circumstances impinge on persons are represented in their effect on the person as an individual subject. The exclusion of 'relationships' became particularly evident during the course of the parliamentary debate where social facts could in this way be taken as subjective ones.

Franklin observes how Baroness Elles's reference to herself as a kinsperson and the relationships this implied located the speaker's experiences as personal (p. 153). In so far as they were mediated by the experiences of the personal witness, social facts were rendered as 'subjective' ones. And they were being brought forward in a context which already contained a very different order of knowledge, the universal and apparently 'objective' facts of embryo development. The power of personal witness lay in the appeal to experiences with which listeners were invited to identify;[27] the weakness of such witness is that its testimony could be marginalised by appeals to a generalised understanding about the future of humanity and of research for the benefit of society that (so the appeal went) should not be held to ransom by individual opinion or experience. As was noted in the previous section, this was facilitated by the way in which it was assumed that the embryo should be included in the debate as an individual entity.

These inclusions and exclusions illuminate a non-relational aspect of the parliamentary debate. Franklin points to how, in evoking different orders of knowledge, the debates could make 'kinship and relationships invisible' (p. 138), for the embryo as a natural entity could seem to be of quite a different order of phenomenon from the legislation that it called into being; indeed, in one sense the authority of legislation was to displace the authority of the natural criteria. In a parallel way, similar displacements affected the perception of social affairs. When social evidence was expressed as 'personal' evidence, it could lose its capacity to refer to relationships and be interpreted as referring to individual circumstances alone. And individual circumstances can be construed (see Chapter 3) as of a quite different order of phenomenon from 'society' at large. Society comes to seem some other domain.

Individual and society are not commensurable. In this ordering of know-ledges, the one can obscure the other. When you see the individual, all you may see are his or her 'personal' preferences or his or her 'personal' cen-tredness. So when in turn the relational is elided with the personal, then *relationships* can lose their 'social' visibility. I have suggested that this possi-bility is prefigured in the kinship constructs of this culture. The cultural analysis of kinship undertaken in these pages, then, does not simply draw on kin relationships to emphasise the 'social' in the social implications of the NRTs; it also suggests just how the social dimension becomes screened off.

There are in turn implications here for the kind of knowledge that 'kinship' brings. Edwards refers to the people she talked with as knowing little about reproductive technology but much about the relationships it was likely to affect: in this they were kinship experts. Expertise necessarily signals both inclusion and exclusion: speakers identify themselves by the semi-autonomy of their expertises (Cannell 1990: 688). Thus legislation will attend to what citizens have in common by right of citizenship, not to the private symbol-ism of every individual person as an individual. It does not, of course, take away the different expertises of individuals with respect to their own situ-ation; it simply bypasses them or makes them irrelevant.[28] Someone trying to pursue the best possible outcome in their own domain, then, will find other claims on the edges of their concerns. The interests of the man or woman who wants to conceive a child are not the same as the interests of the general practitioner who refers them to a clinic nor of the persons who carry out the procedures and whose own concerns barely touch on the specific circumstances of the individuals under treatment.

However, it is not just the obscure which may also appear irrelevant, but the obvious, and not just the idiosyncratic which may appear trivial, but the ubiquitous. At least that is how we might read Baroness Elles's disclaimer about being a simple mother and grandmother. And that is also true of the place of kinship in society. Whatever importance we would like to put on changing conceptualisations of kinship, or however much some people are prepared to talk about it, anthropologists know that in British society, by comparison with many elsewhere, the cultural representations of kinship attribute it a small part in public life. Indeed, public debate on reproductive issues is already constituted as somehow intruding into a private domain. The question, then, is not so much the place of kinship in society as its place in public discourse.

How is kinship represented? It is made to seem both pervasive and restricted, to use C. Harris's words (1990: 3–4). Snowden and Mitchell's (1981) preface to their British study begins with the ubiquitousness of people's experience of family life; the essays in Spallone and Steinberg's (1987) international collection deal with the implications of the NRTs for a range of issues to do with personal identity, autonomy and political power that hardly address kinship at all. Euro-American kinship is represented as both central and marginal – a domain of expertise to which everyone has access *and* one that can be excluded by other considerations. As a consequence, relationships based on kinship are often treated as less than 'socially' significant. We have argued that this is a cultural characteristic of Euro-American kinship thinking, not extraneous but intrinsic to it. Its own discourse problematises the way Euro-Americans conceptualise relationships.

Rather than assert that kinship is important, the studies presented here attempt to show how it is and is not made important, where its presence is an issue or its absence rendered possible. In short, it offers the beginnings of an empirical enquiry that does not take kinship relations for granted but is interested in how kinship itself 'works' culturally as a domain of expertise. What suggested kinship as a domain of enquiry – that it raises issues at the edge of some of the debates that have surrounded the development of reproductive medicine – has thus enhanced our understanding of that domaining effect itself. Enquiry into kinship makes visible or explicit issues that everyone knows are there but which do not always seem relevant to other concerns.

So do problems also turn out to be solutions. Our task has not just been a matter of making kinship appear on the social map. We have to understand why it could ever disappear. And we can suggest that one reason is the way in which the special set of connections that make up Euro-American kinship mediates or contains both relational and non-relational ways of thinking about persons. By virtue of its own constructs, while kinship 'appears' in the former it seems to 'disappear' in the latter. For it recontextualises the order of society and the order of the individual into its own kind of knowledge.

If the effectiveness of Euro-American kinship lies in its mediation of *both* relational and non-relational dimensions of persons, it already exists as a context for the technologies of procreation. The facts of kinship render evident the knowledge that individuals are always brought into the world in the context of relationships. But these facts are known in different ways that must themselves be made evident, and as a matter of empirical enquiry. As an order of knowledge, then, kinship makes and is made by a relational view: it has to take connections into account.

NOTES

1   The differences among ourselves as humans are based on [a small] percentage of our total genetic heritage: a small fraction of 1%. Thus, looking at individual human genomes within our species, common-ness rather than difference is overwhelming. It is this commonness that is our collective heritage and property as human beings. And it is about possible changes in this collective property, which is both a characteristic of the human species and something that is commonly 'owned', that all human beings have a right to be consulted. All of ancestry (past) and all of descendancy (future) are at stake in this lineage that is becoming ever more clearly of rising cosmic significance

(Grobstein 1990: 20).

2 I derive this and several other analytical points from presumptions in the anthropological analysis of symbolic ('representational') practice.
3 The two senses of the idea of relation appear in the statement made by the ILA apropos 'relationships' developing between people already 'related' (see p. 27).
4 I say 'strategy' in order to draw attention to the rhetorical effect. For a recent assessment of the 'textual construction of social reality' and of fram-ing as a rhetorical device, see Atkinson 1990.
5 At least in 'English' Euro-Americanism. Continental European countries vary among themselves in the emphasis put on 'the family' as a public issue. The relative invisibility of such matters would be incomprehensible in France for instance. (It is interesting that one of the few general anthropo-logical works on the Euro-American family to have appeared in recent years is written by a French scholar, see Segalen 1986.)
6 Martin confronts the research strategies of working across social contexts: 'Rather than focus on a bounded setting of any kind, I have deliberately sought out a series of disparate settings in which modal concepts [in this instance] of bodily health are of concern.' I am grateful to Emily Martin for permission to quote from her paper 'Histories of the immune system', pre-sented to the Social Anthropology Department, University of Manchester, 1992.
7 Some of the theoretical background to the formulation of partial connec-tions, and what elsewhere I call the merographic effect of such domaining exercises in Euro-American thinking, can be found in Strathern 1991a and 1992a.
8 From a cultural point of view, such domains are always specific ones, even when the appeal is to common grounding or an apparently higher order of contextualisation. When, in the context of discussing definitions of the per-son, Fagot-Largeault (1990: 153) says that we should attend to the way human cells are disposed of because 'the way we treat human cells is sym-bolic of . . . how we treat humanity', she is evoking a cultural domain of ideas about 'common humanity'. It is a distinct and specific domain that has its own limits. Thus she wants 'the human potential to be respected as human' (the distinctive idea that defines this domain), but respecting the generalised state of humanity does not imply also respecting everything that

human beings have ever done (the domain specifies an area of application that has its limits).

9 They also regulate the unsocialised individual, e.g. 'The family is the place where the first experience of normative order is introduced based upon values associated with the predictability of behaviour' (Snowden *et al.* 1983: 153). On the political ideology that presents the family as carrying 'the whole weight of responsibility for socialization', see McNeil 1991: 233.

10 The point is significant to Cannell's (1990: 672) comparison between certain presuppositions underlying the Warnock Report and the Gillick campaign over contraception. I note that after Rivière 1985 and Wolfram 1989 (also see Wolfram 1987: ch. 11), Cannell's was the first British anthropological commentary that addressed the cultural dimensions of current debates on reproduction.

11 Ethnographic elucidation may be found, for example, in Strathern 1981.

12 The way in which certain interests in the mass media draw on the past to ground the very values they destabilise, as well as on diverse and oppositional scenarios to offset their own messages, is an established theoretical position in cultural studies (cf. Lipsitz quoting the 1970s work of Jürgen Habermas and Stuart Hall).

13 Commentators on the New Right have pointed out the role that the concept of natural, i.e. pre-existing, order plays in its promulgation of morality (e.g. Yoxen 1990; Franklin *et al.* 1991). But that includes the 'naturalness' of persons as individuals who seek to realise their desires.

14 The idea that medical science will in the end be able to do anything is a fantasy that clinicians, among others, have to deal with.

15 Hartouni analyses some of the cultural constructions of motherhood that followed the creation of an American 'orphan embryo' through birth from a brain-dead mother, Odette Henderson. She asks what kind of 'mother' is being described when only the womb is (kept) alive:

> The world held in place by Henderson as brain-dead mother, the world of conventional gender meanings and identities, is precisely the world the new technologies of reproduction destabilize; and, paradoxically, the world these new technologies destabilize is also reinscribed by their ostensible purpose and use as well as by the stories they appear to tell. What, after all, currently legitimates the development of reproductive technologies? They are said to help women realize their maternal nature, their innate need to mother.
>
> (1991: 49)

(My thanks to David Schneider for sending this and other materials.) The general point was observed by Grobstein and Flowers in 1985 when they wrote:

> The initial motivation toward IVF is pro-family – to produce a child for an otherwise incomplete family. But is IVF anti-family in the broader view because it, and its possible variants, will decrease or blur traditional bondings among mother, father and offspring?
>
> (cited in Haimes 1990: 167; emphasis removed)

16 Other people's conservatisms have none the less given anthropology a terminological purchase on developments that seem new in Euro-American eyes. Thus the celebrated distinction between social and biological parenthood as it became variously incorporated into the anthropological canon via Malinowski ('sociological paternity' on the matrilineal Trobriand Islands) and Evans-Pritchard (pater and genitor distinguished by the Nuer) has been recaptured as a kind of wisdom applicable to 'ourselves' that 'other' cultures had already articulated. However, a moment's reflection shows that creating a distinction between parents by splitting apart what was ideally fused (biological and social parenthood in Euro-American culture) is a very different strategy from sustaining the distinctions which the Nuer (say) make between reproduction via individual human beings (the genitor who begets) and via the collective lineage and its cattle (the pater who pays bridewealth). Contemporary accommodations made by the Nuer offer an indigenous commentary on the limitations of both their present and past condition (Hutchinson 1992).

17 Not to speak of various political positions and entrenchments, e.g. patriarchal paradigms (Stolcke 1986) and the racial stereotypes raised by comments reported in Chapter 3.

18 Drawn in the first place from semantic/symbolic anthropology (e.g. Fernandez 1986) but with a long history in the description of social relations. Fernandez specifically addresses the way in which metaphor (image, analogy) moves the perception of experience from the less known to the better known.

19 Metaphor at once effects the connection and keeps distinct the domains it connects (see below). The innovation of meaning is predicated on such 'borrowing' (e.g. Wagner 1972, 1986). On 'substitution' see, for example, Wagner 1978.

20 Most of the time this is done, of course, 'without thinking'. On an explicit evocation of analogy in the House of Lords debate see Strathern 1992b: ch. 7.

21 Cf. Schneider 1968; and the discussion in Strathern 1992a. In Schneider's formulation, persons are relatives in so far as they share substance and observe certain codes of conduct; but relatives are also persons and as persons they act on the basis of their distinct identities. I return to this below.

22 But see the Archbishop of York's distinction between reading history backwards and reading it forwards (p. 150).

23 This is not to say that the 'relating' between mother and child does not begin before birth. I refer to the cultural sense in which even after birth the mother–child pair may be represented as decontextualised 'from society'.

24 Such decontextualising may also be a form of critique directed precisely at 'the understood sense' in the interests of a deliberate recontextualisation of the meanings of family life (for an American example, see Weston 1991).

25 This is not the place for a fuller discussion. However, it should be noted that Schneider stresses the non-kinship criteria that define persons (derived from several domains) by contrast with the single domain of kinship that defines the relative. Our interest in the present study is in the extent to which the English version of Euro-American kinship makes the individual person an artefact of (other persons') kin relations also. Some discussion of the material offered by Schneider and Firth may be found in Strathern 1992a: 82–4.

26 These are the kinds of connections I called merographic (see also Harris 1990: 58).

27 And who could supply in their own minds the wider social contexts from which such experiences might come. But when the context *is* the person (made present in the course of debate as a witness), then all experiences, however apparently incongruent, can also in this culture be related to personal biography.

28 Such screening-out processes render social life 'manageable'. When assisting a person to have a child is a technical feat with its own challenges, the last thing a clinician might want to think about are what the grandparents are going to think. Other domains of knowledge, such as the perspective of the child whose identity is at stake, or of the genetic accuracy of the genealogical record for family medical histories, may be dismissed as irrelevant or as 'other' people's concerns – until, that is, they suddenly present themselves as a request by a client to have children who will also be grandchildren or an attack on medical practice for introducing new fictions into the official record.

Postscript
A relational view

Marilyn Strathern

1993

Can one ask what it would mean to *exclude* kinship from consideration of the new reproductive technologies (NRTs)?

Euro-Americans may think of relationships existing between abstract or inanimate entities, such as 'society' or 'technology'. They also think of them as engaging persons in mutual accord or non-mutual antagonism. As a consequence, people can feel equally empowered by or powerless from relationships that already seem to be in place. Kin relations have a special quality here. They are distinguished from others as relations which are brought into being at the moment of procreation but which from the point of view of the person brought into being are already there.

If, as a consequence, kinship serves for some at least as a vehicle or a mode for talking about limits, and if limits are about relationships, when kinship is disconnected or screened off from other domains of expertise, so we guess is a certain relational approach to the world.

This makes evident anthropology's own relational assumptions. Anthropologists pursue connections between different areas of fact or knowledge about human experience, a comparative exercise whether or not it involves other cultures. They are interested in the particularity or uniqueness that divides one area off from another. We would like to think that between the four studies presented here we have participated in something of that connecting and dividing process. In the course of doing so, the book has addressed two sets of questions. The first is how to evaluate the impact of NRT on kinship relations, and this has been the major part of our concern. The second is how the study itself is to be understood – the diverse contexts in which particular kinds of information become relevant and what kind of information we are providing ourselves. I offer some comments on this second set.

Any study in this field is already participatory, occupies a space in a terrain already occupied, and if it adds a dimension then adds it to others already there. For in a diverse and plural world, however much domains of enquiry appear screened off, or central to themselves, others appear on their margins, and 'other' concerns crop up – with anxiety, criticism or endorsement. New knowledge then appears as a supplement or addition to already-existing knowledge. In that case, to ask why anthropology should have an interest in NRT is to ask in turn what it means to 'add' a further order of facts to what is already known.

In societies beyond Euro-America, anthropologists call themselves participant observers. Their knowledge comes through learning what it might mean to be a participant, much of which is taken up with observing other participants. Yet one cannot really do the same 'at home'. One is already a participant, and to say there are things to learn about one's own society (which is absolutely true) in another sense simply contributes to what one already knows about it (its diversity and plurality). So one has to turn the anthropological exercise around – what has to be learnt is how to observe. Here everyone else is, like oneself, a participant who is also a potential observer. The one thing that anthropologists cannot do is insulate themselves: the one thing they have to do is to acknowledge the way different domains and orders of knowledge impinge on everyone's concerns.

Perhaps in showing how these processes are at work in part of this awkward and complex area, we shall find a way of dealing with the assumptions that differentiate people's experiences and expertises. Differentiation is an artefact of social and cultural life. Not to make the connection would remove us from that. And not to make connections in general would be to endorse a world of insulated problems, to imagine that each issue that arises in the field of reproductive medicine can be separated from others, to be picked off and dealt with in its own terms. Against the specificity which characterises any domain of concern, apprehending the social implications of the NRT must also involve apprehending the way that ideas and practices connect up with one another.

From representation to intervention

Yet 'participation' is altogether too cosy a phrase, and the idea of a natural diversity of viewpoints too neatly sustained by the possibility of their being domained and ordered. It is hardly commensurate with the interventions under study. As Price bluntly states (p. 51), the facilitation of pregnancy is moved into the public domain through the intervention of clinicians, and their facilitations do not simply 'participate' in people's efforts to become parents. They directly affect the way in which these efforts are thought about and carried through. We have already encountered an exaggerated expression of this in (among others) Nicholas Selby's remark that 'giving Nature a helping hand' is fine, but 'trying to create the master race, by fiddling around with genetics' is not (p. 102). The persistent imagery of eugenics does, of course, tell us that there is nothing new in the anxieties or the expectations that intervention provokes.

One significant substitutive effect has accompanied the interventions in the field of reproduction as it has taken shape over the last fifteen years. What is at issue are certain grounding assumptions about processes of human existence. While Euro-Americans may find that they can shed their assumptions as easily as peoples elsewhere have seemingly shed apparently entrenched cosmologies, they may – as has also happened elsewhere – find more being dislodged than they bargained for. Each 'individual' Member of Parliament was invited to make a decision according to his or her con-science. Yet the very diversity that underlies the significance of the indi-vidual, indeed of the cultural pluralism that affords many perspectives, many viewpoints, many opinions, is conventionally underwritten by an understanding of biogenetic diversity. And that for Euro-Americans once defined kinship. In social terms, it is people's position within networks of kin that constitutes their infinite variability, to adapt Edwards' words, even as in genetic terms the randomness of genetic combination is thought to work against the 'standardisation' that Hirsch's acquaintances feared for a market-led environment.

In the future, the market may turn out to be as much an anachronistic reference as fears of a 'master race'. In the meanwhile, it serves to bring to mind a limit of a kind. A market-led world is already a determined one, for variety is determined by pre-existing values. Blue eyes, brown hair, ginger moustache (cf. p. 110), the several comments on race that run through Hirsch's interviews hint at a world of *pre-existing* preferences for certain kinds of people. The idea that follows is that somehow there should be limits on how far these are translated into reality. When interventions of this order seem possible, the only limit on them is further intervention. As a consequence, intervention also creates further uncertainty (cf. Price 1990a). What is 'new' about the NRTs in this sense is the visibility they have given to a sense of infinite regress.

Nowhere has this been more apparent than in the efforts of Parliament. In providing legislation, Parliament sought to provide a set of limits around the possibilities opened up by assisted reproduction. Yet the removal of the *a priori* status of the 'natural facts' upon which kinship reckoning has traditionally been based, and its displacement by the order of technology, in Franklin's words, foregrounded the enabling capacity of scientific progress. The potential to bring new persons and new relation-ships into being imagines a kinship assisted by the removing of limits and enabling of possibilities. In turn, the parliamentarians' dilemmas derive from the assistance they are expected to give to those practitioners who would circumscribe the potential of their craft by ethical and social conventions about what is appropriate.

In the course of that debate, aspects of kinship were 'represented' in various ways: in terms of individuated personhood, of the role of technology in assisting the biological process of conception, and of the meanings to be attached to genetic links. At the same time, the debates intervened by making new conjunctions of ideas visible. Thus Franklin identifies the embryo that was the focus of discussion as an emergent 'kinship' entity of an unfamiliar kind. The embryos being talked about were those whose future (successful [re]implantation) as much as their past (in cases where they were brought into existence through in vitro fertilisation) depended on technological intervention, and whose protection depended on the intervention of legislation. New combinations of knowledge are brought together that create composites every bit as complex as the old view of what makes a kinsperson – the social construction of natural fact – but they are created out of elements perceived as all in some way the outcome of (other) interventions.

When everything seems subject to intervention, then representations come to be seen as interventions too. This is no less true than in the kinds of information such representations are held to rest upon.

> The need is not to remove uncertainty (for that is impossible), but to make it open and positive, rather than covert and manipulative. . . . Unless the issues are argued explicitly, decision-making will be biased to the advantage of the side with the most resources and skills, prejudicing the whole debate.
>
> (Ravetz 1990: 18)

A traditional route to certainty has been through the clarification and division of facts into orders and domains. Thus the first VLA report (1986), in voicing its concern about public misunderstanding about in vitro fertilisation, also noted that this procedure was confused in people's minds with quite different issues such as (the example given) surrogacy. But there is another view. Among the many issues that need to be made explicit is the very way new combinations of information in effect bring together different domains or orders of knowledge. It is no more a 'confusion' on Parliament's part for members debating the ethics of embryo experimentation to inform themselves about the primitive streak than it is a 'confusion' for people to link present and potential possibilities in reproductive medicine. They are simply making certain, present and potential, connections evident.

Bringing together different ideas and thus creating connections or relations between them may lead to misplaced metaphors or errors of association quite as much as it may lead to the illuminating analogy or the additional significant fact. Analogies obscure as well as enlighten. But to denigrate that relational facility would be to denigrate debate or discussion itself.

Rather than dismissing analogy as mere phraseology, we might instead be alert to its cultural effectiveness. In dwelling on the substitutive effects of the way people make connections between different issues that bear on the NRTs, I have also pointed to the power of such representations. For each representation becomes a little intervention. Reproducing the world at the same time alters the way the world is understood; in conserving what they think they already know, people relocate that knowledge. It is thus that Glover *et al.*, for instance, simultaneously conserve and relocate the concept of creation:

> Parents create their children but, beyond this, they are not responsible for their biological characteristics. This may change if it becomes easy to choose the sex or other genetic characteristics of one's child. . . . And being a parent may come to be seen as creating one's children in a much fuller sense than now.
>
> (1989: 56)

From reproduction to procreation

'Reproduction' – that is, replicating an original – enjoys the *double entendre* of representation and having offspring. A reproduction repeats the original, but not in quite the same way. It thus represents it, but in a fresh manner, as we may say offspring represent (reproduce) their parents. The parents are, so to speak, brought back into existence by their child, similar to them though never an exact copy. In never being an exact copy, the child also signals the way variety and diversity are brought into existence. Hence a reproduction always shows its relationship to the original: the old entity is present in new form.

In biology, the term carries its own specific connotations. The extent to which, in the 1980s, reproduction was seized upon to refer to fertility treatments (the new technologies) therefore seemed to need no explanation. Spallone and Steinberg's critical appraisal, sub-titled *The Myth of Reproductive and Genetic Progress* (1987), has a glossary that defines reproductive technology with reference to artificial reproduction techniques; Stanworth's (1987) book takes the fertility reference of 'reproductive technologies' as self-evident. At the same time, these accounts are concerned with representations: with the way that views are presented, the models people use. McNeil (1990) addresses the sociology of technology in this field from this perspective. And in drawing attention to cultural constructions and social consequences, these writers have hoped their own representations of the issue would be interventionist in the public debate. In drawing attention to the word 'procreation', we hope to make such interventionist effect explicit.

Unlike reproduction, 'procreation' is not about the relationship between an original and its offspring/products. Reproduction intimates the completed outcome of a process that leads to further examples being laid beside an original – an original thought brought to mind, a copy of an artefact, children who take after their parents, in short, a species seen again in its 'own kind'. Certainly, the idea of human reproduction is only thinkable in terms of a process that results in children. 'Procreation' has different connotations. Procreation refers to the generative moment, to the act of begetting, to the effectiveness of a capacity. It means to bring into being, to bring forth. Offspring may be implied, but nothing about their similarity to the original. Translated as begetting or propagation, the term tends to be used only of bringing forth young in the biological sense. Here, it has a restricted, indeed old-fashioned air, especially with its connotations of male parenthood: the male progenitor is a procreator. None the less, Gloria de Guy interpreted assisted conception as part of 'the whole field of procreation' (p. 116).

Suppose we exploit some of the characteristics of the term to give it a meaning it does not yet have. To *pro*create is to create in the sense of 'bringing *forth*'. But we could also think of it as creating *on behalf of* another.

This would be a new and artificial etymology. It would, however, draw on an already-existing connotation of the original Latin; *pro* means not just 'for' in the sense of forwards or forth, but also before, in front of, and on behalf of (*OED* 1971). Indeed, in the way in which the Latin preposition has been drawn into English as a prefix, it in any case may refer to a location that is both earlier than and after another, situated in front or behind, anterior or projecting. Its secondary connotations thus point to one thing that supports another, derived from the idea that in being situated in front someone may also *substitute* or *take the place* of and thus act in the stead of the principal [person]. An heir standing in the stead of the parent takes the place of the parent. We might, then, think of the effects of the new technologies in people's views of the world as not so much reproductive as procreative. Rather than raising the question of reproduction, that is, how close to the original the product is, procreation indicates the capacity to create something that will stand in the stead of the original.

Technologies of procreation enable one dimension of Euro-American kinship to work – namely, the extent to which people have always 'worked' to make kinship (Weston 1991: 212). The new work of procreation does something else. Instead of attending to the network of relationships built up after knowledge of biological connection, this new work attends to the biological connections in themselves. It is not just persons who can take one another's places: the same has become true of different aspects of what was once understood as their biogenetic endowment. New capacities stand in the stead of old.

There is, of course, a modernist sense in which description 'stands in the stead' of what it describes. This is representationalism. But our invention of a new connotation out of an old term is meant to draw attention away from the product of description towards how it works. Is the substitute effective? Does it have the capacity to do in the stead of the original? I suspect that this is the postmodernist sense in which technology assists: it substitutes for other cultural capacities. In the case of procreative technology, this is the Euro-American capacity to create kinship.

That we describe the new procedures as technologies carries its own effect. Technology has become a late-twentieth-century metaphor for capacity itself. Whether we think of its enablements or empowerments for better or for ill, the point about technology is that it works. This is true whether it works successfully or not, and why I have laboured the point about intervention. Technological assistance is indeed transformative. What is true about technology is also true about how it is debated, the 'discursive technology' to which Franklin refers. The question that discussion about the NRT raises is what descriptions will work. Here, any mode or enquiry – anthropology among them – has to find a place among several (sometimes competing) discourses. But in finding a place, is its effectiveness to be measured by the extent to which it displaces others? If so, what capacity does it release? Perhaps it works as a new gathering together of issues. Yet it can only work because those issues are already there, as kin relationships are already there as the context for people's procreative endeavours.

The new procreative technologies have opened up possibilities in a field earlier characterised by taken-for-granted assumptions about what is in place. It is no surprise that questions about understanding how things work (representation) should be displaced by questions about how the understandings will work (intervention). Epistemology is more generally displaced by performativity (Lyotard 1984). The success rate with which clinicians are concerned, or questions about the implementation of legislation, are similar to the issue of whose description of the facts will prevail. The only postmodern test is effectiveness.

This is a personal view, and I draw a set of connections that others would not necessarily share. Yet the personal view is also a relational one – and not

simply because it creates a connection between different kinds of knowledge, for such connections may be as misleading as they are helpful – but
because the act of doing so makes explicit (what I would wish to conserve
as) a dimension of social life without which individual persons cannot act
with any effectiveness at all. In realising that one's own views stand in the
stead of other views, other perspectives, persons recreate themselves
through their relationships with other persons.

1998

There is nothing nostalgic in the emphasis which this book has placed on
kinship. Yet to say so is to write against the grain of a culture which regards
kinship as caught up in 'traditional' family life. In this culture, tradition and
family typify the stability of social convention as against 'technology', which
(and it has done so for more than a century now) serves as an apparently
ever-regenerative sign of innovation. There *is* something very persistent and
dogged here. So if at the end of the twentieth century we find that Euro-
Americans are still making kinship in all sorts of ways, it is against a continuing background of concern about how society should intervene in the pace
of technology. Yet one should not make the mistake of imagining that some
bits of the present belong to the past where others do not. The fates of these
interlocking concerns move forward together.

The lapse of five years has underlined – made it even more apparent – the
way in which ideas remain stubbornly locked into one another. Given the
galloping innovations in the field of biomedicine, 'society' still seems the
cart hitched up to the beast 'technology' rather than the other way round.
Ethical and legal guidelines, we are still being told, have to catch up with
technological change. In other words, society is now in the late 1990s, as it
was in the early 1980s when the Warnock Report was commissioned,
imagined as having to keep grasp of a flying creature in front, behind which,
like a rickety two-wheeled chariot, it bumps and lurches along. However,
the cart and horse analogy will not get us very far.

Social science suggests why we might think like that, but also why there is
rather more to it. Lorna Weir and Jasmin Habib (1997) are among many
commentators on the Canadian Royal Commission on New Reproductive
Technologies, launched in the same year as the HFE Bill came to the British
Parliament. Canadian family law, they observe, has evolved in tandem with
a particular kinship system. They use the concept of structural coupling in
order to describe how kinship system and family law each has its own ways
of proceeding and treats the other as outside or beyond itself while at the
same time drawing on it as a source of information in its environment.

Health-care economics and reproductive biology is another linked example.[1] The term 'structural coupling' comes from writings on complex systems which need not detain us here, and especially though not exclusively (in this case) on institutions within a state framework. The point is that specific domains of social life may find themselves hooked into other specific domains, while each also pursues its own semi-autonomous trajectory. So from one point of view kinship and family law travel in tandem; from another they are like figure and ground spinning through separate revolutions. Look through the chariot wheels from the side. The wheels will be turning round together but the revolution of one set of spokes will be superimposed on the other. Kinship and family law each appears with its own distinct configuration of elements against the separately moving yet hooked-up background of the other. But while sometimes the background will take a distinct shape (another 'domain' or 'system'), at other times it will appear more diffuse, like the moving landscape glimpsed through both sets of spokes. Although 'environment' is a technical term[2] in Weir and Habib's model, we can keep with the image of figure and (back)ground, provided we realise neither stays still.

Taking the context of people's actions and decisions as an environment in this sense points to a crucial property. It describes a limit. That is, the difference between the phenomenon and its environment establishes a boundary between them. Like technology and society, assisted conception and kinship relations form fields, each of which seems at once to challenge and limit the other. Perhaps this helps elucidate the persistently paradoxical nature of *intervention*, for at the point at which advice or expertise is taken from one field or domain to illuminate another it appears already to have been translated into the terms and conventions of the receiving domain.

Here we can appreciate some of the problems of representation which have arisen in our studies: questions about who acts on behalf of whom, or who speaks for whom, come into view when social identities and capacities that 'belong' to one domain become the environment for another that at once draws them in and changes them, in order to make them relevant for itself. There is a 'procreative' (producing on behalf of another) effect here.

If technology and society have been coupled in debate, there have been other persistent and apparently successful couplings among various actors. Thus, where it has not been steered by clinicians, most public discussion of the NRTs in the UK and Europe has been steered by moral philosophers and ethicists. Now to date the weight of the coupling between ethicists on the one hand and policy discussion about reproductive medicine on the other has been towards illuminating the largely non-relational consequences of novel medical practices. Fascinating and important as these contributions are, they also come up against inevitable limitations of understanding.

These limitations are reached as soon as one asks about the (environment of) social consequences. Problems are all too often – there are notable exceptions[3] – instead addressed in terms of the quantity of harm or benefit likely to ensue; although in a limited way this approach tries to imagine the impact that one person's actions will have on another, the register remains a calculation of individual gain or loss. This occludes both the social relationships set up by the procedures under discussion and the pre-existing relationships which influence and are influenced by them.

Yet what may be ignored in the course of these arguments cannot be ignored by the people who seek out or are offered the procedures. If we remain puzzled as to why solutions continue to create problems, then perhaps here is an environment which needs to be brought into view. Social relationships *are* the social reality – context and environment – within which people act according to ethical decisions. However, the general social environment is not like these other couplings – rather, it is the context out of which specific couplings emerge which obscure the larger field, as for example, society (minus technology) and technology do. Another example: out of diverse social relations, this book has been concerned largely with those of kinship, and less with the chains of relations involved in the administration of treatments.

One of the problems with structural coupling as such is that it locks together ideas or domains of actions as distinct fields of reference in such a way as to also occlude the extent to which they already participate in one another. So 'society' is asked to intervene in 'technology' as though technology were not already a social process and as though society were not already, in Latour's memorable phrase, technology made durable. You cannot imagine either figure or ground without the other. Persons, too, are part of the new technologies which they may see as bearing in on them with greater or lesser implication for social relationships.

Here the anthropologist's interest in kinship is of a piece with other concerns in social science which have been gathering over the last five years. I give three examples; they point in one interesting direction. These social scientists wish to make a point about what on the surface is a simple and rather obvious fact: the increase in the number of actors brought about through technological intervention in the reproductive process. Now from one point of view there is nothing new in this observation. There have been many commentaries on the intervention of medical agents in assisting conception as well as birth. The addition of potential parents through gamete donation and surrogacy arrangements may add a sense of further and increasing complexity. Frequently this social complexity is felt to get in the way of the 'simple' process of having a baby, bringing in complications such as the shadowy, anonymous donor lurking on the edges of the new family.

What these writers draw to our attention is the fact that each additional procedure increases the number of social actors, and that this introduces shifts of control and interests. Each technological innovation creates, and is created by, possibilities for new dependencies.[4] In reproductive medicine the interests are to do with claims to social relationships. Some of these concern the exercise of expert knowledge (clinician, counsellor), while others concern the child as a social being or the exercise of choice.

The embryo fertilised in vitro and then suspended in frozen storage is the subject of Simone Bateman Novaes' and Tania Salem's (1998) contribution to a volume on 'the future' of reproduction. They wish to sidestep philosophical and legal argument about the status of the embryo in order to focus on the social context within which this entity exists. Assisted conception increases what they call 'the complexity of the network' surrounding the embryo; it also raises questions about how the network participants and their various arguments should be ranked. In this sense, technology has multiplied the number and type of actors involved in the conception. One focus of these persons' activity is the embryo, itself not so much an actor as an actant[5] that compels others to speak for it. Here it becomes evident that the actors bring further networks into play, for, as the authors go on to depict it, they compete among themselves for prevalence in deciding an embryo's fate, thus ultimately quarrelling over which of them is best qualified to speak on its behalf (cf. Callon 1986).[6] Others take it on themselves to speak for society. In effect, an outcome of the lengthening chain of actors is further debate (in this case the debate is over the relative rights of mother and child). This is what the technology has, so to speak, also produced. As the two authors note, it is apparently increased technical mastery over the conditions of medical treatment which is changing the way decision-making is distributed or delegated among the actors in the embryo's network.

Speaking on behalf the child is central to the kinds of claims that Erica Haimes (1998) examines in her account of the child born through donor insemination (DI). She is concerned, in her words, not just with how the child is represented in the sense of imagined but how it is represented in the sense of being given a voice through the voice of others. This second type of representation is epitomised in the concept of the welfare of the child, a kind of passage point for the alignment of interests. She notes how the range of representatives, those who do speak on behalf of the child, fluctuates at different points. Thus the person at the end of treatment is regarded as the successful outcome of DI assistance, and at this point the network alters shape, the recipient of treatment becoming a parent to a child and the clinician receding into facilitator, as parts of the network become concealed from one another. One recurrent debate in this area is over the relative advantages of anonymity, and behind the clinicians' withdrawal the identity of the donor can remain hidden. Haimes is concerned to show that the DI child, so often regarded as a product of technology, is simultaneously a product of social relations and social processes. Fascination with techno-logical process occludes the lengthening chain of actors/actants, human and non-human, which also sustains it. It is not just a matter of numbers: people are operating here at different levels and with different priorities to promote.

Finally, let me return to Weir, who argues that feminist critique of devel-opments in reproductive medicine could do well to shift from focusing on 'the technology' to foregrounding those practices of governance so often left in the background. The management of interests is at once linked to 'technology' and has its own trajectory. This would move enquiry 'away from critical and reactive commentaries on technical innovations to a very thick description of the administrative and discursive construction of preg-nancy' (1996: 389). Her own argument locates a focus for administrative decision-making in a particular definition of pregnancy: the condition of pregnancy is defined as a condition of risk and must be managed. If risk management becomes the passage point through which actors find their arguments squeezed, then debate concerns the degree of regulation com-patible with individual freedom. Again, with technology has come a length-ening of the chains: present-day risk management has to go through assessment of the biomedical procedures themselves.[7] Actors increase (the number of) actors: it is this human mobilisation which in turn gives techno-logical intervention part of its runaway character.

Numerous actors vie for precedence, then, as Bateman and Salem put it, in deciding the fate of the embryo – or the IVF child or the pregnant woman. But these entities (frozen embryo, DI child, assisted pregnancy) are not the only objects created through the ensuing discourse, and it is not only tech-nological process that involves a lengthening, and ever more complex, chain of actors. Consider the child of donated gametes. Regardless of any ambiguity or doubt about human choices in the matter, or whether the outcome is secrecy or public knowledge, when one separates out the role played by medical technology, 'the technology' seems to be succeeding anyway (the child is born); it remains enabling, appears almost to have a life of its own. Once we have seen that, a counterpoint becomes visible. The terms in which the debate over the particular ambiguities or choices is conducted may well have preceded these particular interventions, itself stemming from longstanding ideas about family life or changing adoption procedures, or whatever. In this sense, it is *the debate* which has an independent life of its own.[8] Indeed there is often a well-rehearsed air to the way in which issues to do with the personhood of the embryo, the welfare of the child, donor anonymity, or the autonomy of the pregnant woman for that matter, are pursued. In particular situations of conflict or policy direct-ive, each problem offers a significant 'passage point' for the actors. Yet the accompanying discourses may well continue to exist after the issue of the moment has receded, and thus in effect exist as objects with their own networks of actants, including other sources of enduring debate: from the network of arguments over 'the embryo' to the network of arguments over 'the autonomy of the mother'.

Like technology, debate increases the number and complexity of the social interests that are part of it. The challenge will be not to couple decision-making to any one set of interests. But this may well seem to go against the grain of a culture for whom regular couplings are ways of reducing complexity, ways of at once making things manageable and gov-ernable, and ways of explaining itself (technology) to itself (society).

NOTES

1 There are 'multiple sites of structural coupling involving the state'. For example:

> Public health care was historically structurally coupled with obstetrics and gynaecology, but the ongoing displacement of obstetrics and gynaecology by the rapidly changing subdiscipline of reproductive biology, which is in turn structurally coupled with biotechnology, introduces new sets of options for public health care (1997: 146).

2 In so far as it is a source of information, one social system can serve as an environment for another. Technically speaking, a system or domain, in turn, is defined by the translation work it does on its environment.
3 As reflected in the interests of Brenda Almond, to take one example, who is Director of the Social Values Research Centre at the University of Hull.
4 More neutrally, for Latour (1993: 108), some of the 'power' of technology lies in its multiplication of the non-humans ('objects') enrolled in human enterprises, the greater the number of objects the greater the number of (human) subjects.
5 While I have referred to aspects of what John Law (e.g. 1994: 100–4) calls actor network theory in the work of Latour, Callon and others, I make idio-syncratic usage of the terms 'actant' and 'actor'. 'Actants' are any entities, human or non-human, who compel others to take action, as we may say that medical instruments can only be effective if people work them properly. I use the more familiar 'actor' when only human actants are involved.
6 Callon is interested in the power process ('*intéressement*') by which actors attempt to stabilise the identity of other actors – human or non-human – in order to enrol them into their project. Who speaks for whom, and thus who represents whom, becomes a crucial gambit in this process; another is the

creation of definitive passage points on which actors force others to focus, e.g. in the case of arguments over embryo research the point at which its person-like qualities may be said to appear (see Mulkay 1997: ch. 7).

7 A process which informed the outcome of the Canadian Royal Commission on the New Reproductive Technologies with its emphasis on evidence-based medicine to control health-care provision (see *Proceed with Care: The Final Report of the Royal Commission in New Reproductive Technologies*, Ottawa: Canada Communications Group, 1993).

8 See, for example, Haimes (1992) on debate over gamete donation.

Bibliography

Abdalla, H. (1990) 'Oocyte donation results', *IVF Congress Magazine 1990*, 10.
—— (1996) 'A national oocyte donation society is needed', *Human Reproduction*, 11, 2355–6.
Abdalla, H. and Studd, J.W. (1989) 'Egg donation and medical ethics', *British Medical Journal*, 299, 120.
Abrahams, R. (1990), 'Plus ça change, plus c'est la même chose? [Organ donation and kinship], *Australian Journal of Anthropology*, spec. issue, 'On the generation and maintenance of person', W. Shapiro (ed.), 1, 131–46.
Anderson, D.C. (1987) 'Licensing work on IVF and related procedures', *Lancet*, 1, 1373.
Archbishop of Canterbury's Commission (1948) *Artificial Human Insemination: The Report of a Commission Appointed by His Grace the Archbishop of Canterbury*, London: Society for the Promotion of Christian Knowledge.
Ardener, E. (1987) '"Remote areas": some theoretical considerations', in A. Jackson (ed.), *Anthropology at Home*, London: Tavistock.
Atkinson, P. (1990) *The Ethnographic Imagination*, London: Routledge.
Ballard, R. (1990) 'Migration and kinship: the differential effect of marriage rules on the processes of Punjabi migration to Britain', in C. Clarke (ed.), *South Asians Overseas*, Cambridge: Cambridge University Press.
Baldwin, T. *et al.* (1996) *Convergence: Integrating Media, Information and Communication*, London: Sage.
Bartholet, E. (1993) *Family Bonds: Adoption and the Politics of Parenting*, New York: Houghton Mifflin.
Bateman Novaes, S. and Salem, T. (1998) 'Embedding the embryo', in J. Harris and C. Erin (eds), *The Future of Reproduction: Ethics, Choice and Regulation*, Oxford: Oxford University Press.
Battaglia, D. (1995) 'Fear of selfing in the American cultural imaginary or "you are never alone with a clone"', *American Anthropologist* 97 (4): 672–678.
Bell, V. (1991) *Health, Harm or Happy Families? Knowledges of Incest in Twentieth-century Parliamentary Debate*, Paper presented to British Sociological Association, Health and Society Conference, Manchester.

Bennett, S.J., Parsons, J.H. and Bolton, V.N. (1989) 'Two embryo transfer', *Lancet*, 11, 215.

Benson, S. (1981) *Ambiguous Ethnicity: Interracial Families in London*, Cambridge: Cambridge University Press.

Berger, D.M., Eisen, A., Shuber, J. and Doody, K.F. (1986) 'Psychological patterns in donor insemination couples', *Canadian Journal of Psychiatry*, 31, 818–22.

Bhachu, P. (1985) *Twice Migrants: East African Sikh Settlers in Britain*, London: Tavistock.

Biggers, J.D. (1981) 'In vitro fertilisation and embryo transfer in human beings', *New England Journal of Medicine*, 34, 336–42.

Bolton, V., Golombok, S., Cook, R., Bish, A. and Rust, J. (1991) 'A comparative study of attitudes towards donor insemination and egg donation in recipients, potential donors and the public', *Journal of Psychosomatic Obstetrics and Gynaecology*, 12, 217–28.

Botting, B.J., Macfarlane, A.J. and Price, F.V. (1990) *Three, Four and More: A Study of Triplets and Higher Order Births*, London: Her Majesty's Stationery Office.

Bouquet, M. (1993) *Reclaiming English Kinship: Portuguese Refractions on British Kinship Theory*, Manchester: Manchester University Press.

Braude, P. and Johnson, M. (1990) 'The embryo in contemporary medical science', in G. Dunstan (ed.), *The Human Embryo: Aristotle and the Arabic and European Traditions*, Exeter: University of Exeter Press.

Braude, P., Johnson, M.H. and Aitken, R.J. (1990) 'Human Fertilisation and Embryo Bill goes to report stage', *British Medical Journal*, 300, 1410–12.

British Agencies for Adoption and Fostering (BAAF) (1990) 'Human Fertilisation and Embryology Bill: Joint Briefing paper from British Agencies for Adoption and Fostering and British Association of Social Workers'.

Brody, E.M. (1987) 'Reproduction without sex, but with the doctor', *Law, Medicine and Health Care*, 15, 152–5.

Bromham, D., Dalton, M.E. and Jackson, J.C. (eds) (1990) *Philosophical Ethics in Reproductive Medicine*, Manchester: Manchester University Press.

Burton, B., Chan, C.L.K., Puzko, Z. and Wood, E.D. (1986) 'Attitudes towards oocyte and embryo donation and disposal', *Australian and New Zealand Journal of Obstetrics and Gynaecology*, 26, 304–8.

Callon, M. (1986) 'Some elements of the sociology of translation: domestication of the scallops and the fishermen of St Brieuc Bay', in J. Law (ed.), *Power, Action and Belief: A New Sociology of Knowledge*, London: Routledge.

Cannell, F. (1990) 'Concepts of parenthood: the Warnock Report, the Gillick debate, and modern myths', *American Ethnologist*, 17, 4, 667–86.

Carsten, J. (1995) 'The substance of kinship and the heat of the hearth: feeding, personhood and relatedness among Malays in Pulau Langkawi' *American Ethnologist* 22: 223–241.

—— (1997) *The Heat of the Hearth: The Process of Kinship in a Malay Fishing Community*, Oxford: Oxford University Press.

—— (ed.) (forthcoming) *Cultures of Relatedness: New Approaches to the Study of Kinship*, Cambridge: Cambridge University Press.

Charsley, S.R. (1991) *Rites of Marrying: The Wedding Industry in Scotland*, Manchester: Manchester University Press.

Cohen, A.P. (1987) *Whalsay: Symbol, Segment and Boundary in a Shetland Island Community*, Manchester: Manchester University Press.

Collier, J. and Yanagisako, S. (eds) (1987) *Gender and Kinship: Towards a Unified Analysis*, Stanford: Stanford University Press.

Contrepas, C. (1989) 'Information before pregnancy', *Multiple Births Foundation Newsletter*, 5, 2.

Craft, I. (1997), 'An "inconvenience allowance" would solve the egg shortage', *British Medical Journal*, 314, 1400–1.

Crosbie, P. (1992) 'Test tube baby at 50', *Daily Express*, 10 March, 5.

Cussins, C. (1996) 'Ontological choreography: agency through objectification in infertility clinics', *Social Studies of Science*, 26, 575–610.

—— (1998) 'Producing reproduction: techniques of normalization and naturalization in infertility clinics', in S. Franklin and H. Ragoné, (eds), *Reproducing Reproduction: Kinship, Power and Technological Innovation*, Philadelphia, PA: University of Pennsylvania Press.

Dawson, K.J., Rutherford, A.J., Margam, R.A., Winston, R.M.L. (1991) 'Reducing triplet pregnancies following in-vitro fertilisation', *Lancet*, 337, 1543–4.

Delaney, C. (1986) 'The meaning of paternity and the virgin birth debate', *Man*, 21, 494–513.

Department of Health and Social Security (1984) *Report of the Committee of Inquiry into Human Fertilisation and Embryology* (The Warnock Report), Cmnd. 9314, London: Her Majesty's Stationery Office.

Derom, C., Derom, R., Vlietinck, R., Van Den Berge, H. and Theiry, M. (1987) 'Increased monozygotic twinning after ovulation induction', *Lancet*, 1, 1236–8.

Dickenson, D.L. (1997) 'Procuring gametes for research and therapy: the argument for unisex altruism – a response to Donald Evans', *Journal of Medical Ethics*, 23, 93–5.

Dunstan, G.R. (1990) 'The moral status of the human embryo', in D. Bromhan, M.E. Dalton and J.C. Jackson (eds), *Philosophical Ethics in Reproductive Medicine*, Manchester: Manchester University Press.

Dyson, A. (1990) 'At Heaven's command? The churches, theology and experiments on embryos', in A. Dyson and J. Harris (eds), *Experiments on Embryos*, London: Routledge.

Edelmann, R.G. and Golombok, S. (1989) 'Stress and reproductive failure', *Journal of Reproductive and Infant Psychology*, 7, 79–86.

Edwards, J. (1990) 'Ordinary people: a study of factors affecting communication in the provision of services', PhD, Manchester University.

Edwards, J. and Strathern, M. (forthcoming) 'Including our own', in J. Carsten (ed.), *Cultures of Relatedness: New Approaches to the Study of Kinship*.

Edwards, R.G. (1985) 'In-vitro fertilisation and embryo replacement: opening lecture', *Annals of the New York Academy of Science*, 442, 375–80.

Edwards, R.G., Mettler, L. and Walters, D.E. (1986) 'Identical twins and in vitro fertilisation', *Journal of In Vitro Fertilisation and Embryo Transfer*, 3, 114–17.

Edwards, R.G. and Steptoe, P. (1980) *A Matter of Life: The Story of a Medical Breakthrough*, London: Hutchinson.

Elliot, F.R. (1986) *The Family: Change or Continuity?* London: Macmillan Education.

Fagot-Largeault, A. (1990) 'The notion of the potential human being', in D.R. Bromham, M.E. Dalton and J.C. Jackson (eds), *Philosophical Ethics in Reproductive Medicine*, Manchester: Manchester University Press.

Fernandez, J.W. (1986) *Persuasions and Performances: The Play of Tropes in Culture*, Bloomington, IN: Indiana University Press.

Finch, J. (1989) *Family Obligations and Social Change*, Cambridge: Polity Press.

Fincham, E., Brinsden, P. and Craft, I. (1989) 'Parents' response to a question-naire on assisted reproduction treatment', *Ethical Problems in Reproductive Medicine*, 1, 25–7.

Firth, R., Hubert, J. and Forge, A. (1969) *Families and their Relatives. Kinship in a Middle-Class Sector of London*, London: Routledge & Kegan Paul.

Fishel, S. and Webster, J. (1987) 'IVF and associated techniques: whom can we believe?', *Lancet*, II, 273.

Ford, N. (1988) *When Did I Begin? Conceptions of the Human Individual in History, Philosophy and Science*, Cambridge: Cambridge University Press.

Franklin, S. (1990) 'Deconstructing "desperateness": the social construction of infertility in popular representations of new reproductive technologies', in M. McNeil *et al.* (eds), *The New Reproductive Technologies*, London: Macmillan.

—— (1991) 'Fetal Fascinations: new dimensions to the medical-scientific con-struction of fetal personhood', in S. Franklin, C. Lury and J. Stacey (eds), *Off-Centre: Feminism and Cultural Studies*, London: Harper-Collins Academic.

—— (1992) 'Contested Conceptions: a cultural account of science and procreation', PhD, Birmingham University.

—— (1997) *Embodied Progress: A Cultural Account of Assisted Conception*, London: Routledge.

Franklin, S., Lury, C. and Stacey, J. (1991) 'Feminism, Marxism and Thatcher-ism', in S. Franklin, C. Lury and J. Stacey (eds), *Off-Centre: Feminism and Cultural Studies*, London: HarperCollins Academic.

Fraser, L. (1987) 'Sisters share test tube joy of twin girls', *Mail on Sunday*, 8 November, 17.

Gellner, E. (1987) *The Concept of Kinship and Other Essays on Anthropological Method and Explanation*, Oxford: Basil Blackwell.

Ginsburg, F. (1989) *Contested Lives: The Abortion Debate in an American Community*, Boston: Beacon Press.

Glover, J. *et al.* (1989) *Fertility and the Family*, The Glover Report on the Reproductive Technologies to the European Commission, London: Fourth Estate.

Goldthorpe, J.E. (1987) *Family Life in Western Societies: A Historical Sociology of Family Relationships in Britain and North America*, Cambridge: Cambridge University Press.

Goody, E. (1982) *Parenthood and Social Reproduction*, Cambridge: Cambridge University Press.

Goody, J. (1983) *The Development of the Family and Marriage in Europe*, Cambridge: Cambridge University Press.

Gosden, R.C. (1985) 'Maternal age: a major factor affecting the prospects and outcome of pregnancy', *Annals of New York Academy of Science*, 442, 45–57.

Grobstein, C. (1990) 'Genetic manipulation and experimentation', in D.R. Bromham, M.E. Dalton and J.C. Jackson (eds), *Philosophical Ethics in Reproductive Medicine*, Manchester: Manchester University Press.

Gunning, J. and English, V. (1993) *Human In Vitro Fertilisation: A case study in the regulation of medical innovation*, Aldershot: Dartmouth Publishing Company.

Haimes, E. (1990) 'Recreating the family? Policy considerations relating to the "new" reproductive technologies', in M. McNeil *et al.* (eds), *The New Reproductive Technologies*, London: Macmillan.

—— (1991) 'Gender, gametes and the new reproductive technologies', paper presented at the British Sociological Association Annual Conference, Manchester.

—— (1992) 'Gamete donation and the social management of genetic origins', in M. Stacey (ed.), *Changing Human Reproduction: Social Science Perspectives*, London: Sage.

—— (1998) 'Changing representations of 'the child', in K. Daniels and E. Haimes (eds), *International Social Science Perspectives on Donor Insemination*, Cambridge: Cambridge University Press.

Hall, S. (1997) 'The centrality of culture: notes on the cultural revolution of our time', in K. Thompson (ed.), *Media and Cultural Regulation*, London: Sage.

Handler, R. (ed.) (1995) *Schneider on Schneider: The Conversion of the Jews and Other Anthropological Stories*, Durham, NC: Duke University Press.

Hansen, J. (1986) 'Older maternal age and pregnancy outcome: a review of the literature', *Obstetrics and Gynaecology Survey*, 41, 726–34.

Harris, C.C. (1990) *Kinship*, Milton Keynes: Open University Press.

Harris, J. (1992) *Wonder Woman and Superman: The Ethics of Human Biotechnology*, Oxford: Oxford University Press.

Hartouni, V. (1991) 'Containing women: reproductive discourse in the 1980s', in C. Penley and A. Ross (eds), *Technoculture*, Minneapolis, MN: University of Minnesota Press.

Harvey, D. (1989) *The Condition of Postmodernity*, Oxford: Blackwell.

Hayden, C. (1998) 'A biodiversity sampler for the millennium', in S. Franklin and H. Ragoné (eds), *Reproducing Reproduction: Kinship, Power and Technological Innovation*, Philadelphia: University of Pennsylvania Press.

Heilmreich, S. (1998) 'Replicating Reproduction in Artificial Life: Or, the essence of life in the age of virtual electronic reproduction', in S. Franklin and H. Ragoné (eds), *Reproducing Reproduction: Kinship, Power and Technological Innovation*, Philadelphia: University of Pennsylvania Press.

Hirsch, E. (1992) 'The long term and the short term of domestic consumption: an ethnographic case study', in R. Silverstone and E. Hirsch (eds), *Consuming Technologies*, London: Routledge.

—— (1998a) 'Bound and unbound entities: reflections on the ethnographic perspectives of anthropology vis-à-vis media and cultural studies', in F. Hughes-Freeland (ed.), *Ritual, Performance, Media*, London: Routledge.

—— (1998b) 'New technologies and domestic consumption', in C. Geraghty and D. Lusted (eds), *The Television Studies Book*, London: Arnold.

—— (1998c) 'Domestic appropriations: multiple contexts and relational limits in the home-making of Greater Londoners', in N. Rapport and A. Dawson (eds), *Migrants of Identity: Perceptions of Home in a World of Movement*, Oxford: Berg.

Holy, L. (1996) *Anthropological Perspectives on Kinship*, London: Pluto Press.

Home Office and Scottish Home Department (1960) *Report of the Departmental Committee on Human Artificial Insemination* (The Feversham Report), Cmnd. 1105, London: Her Majesty's Stationery Office.

Hull, M.G.R., Glazener, C., Kelly, N., Conway, D., Foster, P., Watt, E. and Desai, K. (1985) 'Population study of causes, treatment and outcome of infertility', *British Medical Journal*, 219, 1693–7.

Human Fertilisation and Embryology Authority (1991) *Code of Practice: Explanation*, London: HFEA.

—— (1998) *Consultation on the Implementation of Withdrawal of Payments to Donors*, London: HFEA.

Hutchinson, S. (1992) 'The cattle of money and the cattle of girls among the Nuer, 1930–83', *American Ethnologist*, 19, 294–316.

Inhorn, M. (1994) *Quest for Conception: Gender, Infertility, and Egyptian Medical Traditions*, Philadelphia, PA: University of Pennysylvania Press.

—— (1996) *Infertility and Patriarchy: the cultural politics of gender and family life in Egypt*, Philadelphia, PA: University of Pennsylvania Press.

Inhorn, M. and Van Balen, F. (eds) (1999) *Interpreting Infertility: Childlessness, Gender, and the New Reproductive Technologies in Global Perspective*, Berkeley, CA: University of California Press.

Interim Licensing Authority (1990a) *The Fifth Report of the Interim Licensing Authority for Human In Vitro Fertilisation and Embryology*, London: ILA.

—— (1990b) *Egg Donation: Your Questions Answered*, London: ILA.

—— (1991) *The Sixth Report of the Interim Licensing Authority for Human In Vitro Fertilisation and Embryology*, London: ILA.

Johnson, M.H. (1997) 'The culture of unpaid and voluntary egg donation should be strengthened', *British Medical Journal*, 313, 1401–02.

Kennedy, I. (1988) 'What is a medical decision?', in I. Kennedy, *Treat Me Right: Essays in Medical Law and Ethics*, Oxford: Clarendon Press.

Kerr, A., Cunningham-Burley, S. and Amos, A. (1997) 'The new genetics: professionals' discursive boundaries', *Sociological Review*, 45, 279–303.

Kahn, S. (1997) 'Reproducing Jews: the social uses and cultural meanings of the new reproductive technologies in Israel', Doctoral dissertation submitted to the Department of Anthropology, Harvard University (forthcoming from Duke University Press).

Kolata, G. (1997) *The Road to Dolly and the Path Ahead*, London: Allen Lane, Penguin Press.

La Fontaine, J.S. (1985) 'Anthropological perspectives on the family and social change', *The Quarterly Journal of Social Affairs*, 1, 29–56.

—— (1988) 'Child sex abuse and the incest taboo: practical problems and theoretical issues', *Man*, 23, 1–18.

—— (1990) *Child Sex Abuse*, Oxford: Polity Press.

Latour, B. (1993) *We Have Never Been Modern* (trans. C. Porter), London: Harvester Wheatsheaf.

Law, J. (1994) *Organizing Modernity*, Oxford: Blackwell.

Leach, E. (1966) 'Virgin birth', *Proceedings of the Royal Anthropological Institute*, 39–49.

Leeton, J., Trounson, A. and Wood, C. (1984) 'The use of donor eggs and embryos in the management of infertility', *Australian and New Zealand Journal of Obstetrics and Gynaecology*, 24, 265–70.

Leeton, J. and Harman, J. (1986) 'Attitudes towards egg donation of thirty-four infertile women who donated during their in vitro fertilisation treatment', *Journal of In Vitro Fertilisation and Embryo Transfer*, 3, 374–8.

Lefort, C. (1986) *The Political Forms of Modern Society* (trans. and introduced by J.B. Thompson), Oxford: Polity Press.

Leiblum, S.R., Kemmann, E. and Takse, L. (1989) 'Attitudes toward multiple births', Paper presented at the 9th International Congress of Psychosomatic Obstetrics and Gynaecology, Amsterdam, 28–31 May.

Levene, M.I. (1986) 'Grand multiple pregnancies and demand for neonatal intensive care', *Lancet*, 2, 347–8.

—— (1991) 'Assisted reproduction and its implications for paediatrics', *Archives of Diseases in Childhood*, 66, 1–3.

Lilford, R.J. and Dalton, M.E. (1987) 'Effectiveness of treatment for infertility', *British Medical Journal*, 295, 155–6.

Lipsitz, G. (1986) 'The meaning of memory: family, class, and ethnicity in early network television programmes', *Cultural Anthropology*, 1, 355–87.

Lukes, S. (1973) *Emile Durkheim*, London: Penguin Books.

Lutjen, P., Trounson, A., Leeton, J., Findlay, J., Wood, C. and Renou, P. (1984) 'The establishment and maintenance of pregnancy using in vitro fertilisation and embryo donation in a patient with premature ovarian failure', *Nature*, 307, 174.

Lyotard, J-F. (1984 [1979]) *The Postmodern Condition: A Report on Know-ledge* (trans. C. Bennington and B. Massumi), Manchester: Manchester University Press.

Macfarlane, A.J., Johnson, A. and Bower, P. (1990) 'Disabilities and health problems in childhood', in B.J. Botting, A.J. Macfarlane and F.V. Price (eds), *Three, Four and More: A Study of Triplets and Higher Order Births*, London: Her Majesty's Stationery Office, 153–60.

McKie, R. (1988) 'Twins disprove "medical first"', *Observer*, 28 February, 2.

McNeil, M. (1990) 'Reproductive technologies: a new terrain for the sociology of technology', in M. McNeil *et al.* (eds), *The New Reproductive Technologies*, London: Macmillan.

—— (1991) 'Making and not making the difference: the gender politics of Thatcherism', in S. Franklin, C. Lury and J. Stacey (eds), *Off-Centre: Feminism and Cultural Studies*, London: Harper Collins Academic.

McNeil, M., Varcoc, I. and Yearley, S. (eds) (1990) *The New Reproductive Technologies*, London: Macmillan.

McWhinnie, A.M. (1967) *Adopted Children: How they Grow Up. A Study of their Adjustment as Adults*, London: Routledge and Kegan Paul.

—— (1986) 'AID and infertility', *Adoption and Fostering*, 10, 16–18.

Malinowski, B. (1927) *The Father in Primitive Society*, New York: W.W. Norton.

—— (1930) 'Parenthood: the basis of social structure', in V. F. Calverton and D. Schmalhausen (eds), *The New Generation: The Intimate Problems of Modern Parents and Children*, London: Allen and Unwin.

Marcus, G. (1995) 'Ethnography in/of the world system: the emergence of multi-sited ethnography', *Annual Review of Anthropology*, 24: 95–117.

Mathieson, D. (1986) 'Infertility services in the NHS: what's going on?', Report prepared for Frank Dobson, MP, House of Commons.

Medical Research International Society for Assisted Reproductive Technology, The American Fertility Society (1991) 'In vitro fertilization-embryo transfer (IVF-ET) in the United States: 1989 results from the IVF-ET registry', *Fertility and Sterility*, 55, 14–23.

Miller, D. (1987) *Material Culture and Mass Consumption*, Oxford: Blackwell.

Mills, J. (1991) *Womanwords*, London: Virago.

Montagu, A. (1937) *Coming into Being Among the Australian Aborigines*, London: Routledge and Kegan Paul.

Morgan, D. and Lee, R.G. (1991) *Blackstone's Guide to the Human Fertilisation and Embryology Act 1990: Abortion and Embryo Research*, London: Blackstone Press.

Morgan, L.M. (1989) 'When does life begin? A cross-cultural perspective on the personhood of fetuses and young children', in E. and J. Prescott (eds), *Abortion Rights and Fetal Personhood*, Long Beach, CA: Centerline Press.

Morse, C.A. and Van Hall, E.V. (1987) 'Psychosocial aspects of infertility: a review of current concepts', *Journal of Psychosomatic Obstetrics and Gynaecology*, 6, 157–64.

MRC Working Party on Children Conceived by In-Vitro Fertilisation (1990),

'Births in Great Britain resulting from assisted conception, 1978–87', *British Medical Journal*, 300, 1229–33.

Mugford, M. (1990) 'The cost of a multiple birth', in B. J. Botting, A. J. Macfarlane and F. V. Price (eds), *Three, Four and More: A Study of Triplets and Higher Order Births*, London: Her Majesty's Stationery Office, 205–17.

Mulkay, M. (1997) *The Embryo Research Debate: Science and the Politics of Reproduction*, Cambridge: Cambridge University Press.

National Perinatal Statistics Unit (1990) *IVF and GIFT Pregnancies: Australia and New Zealand 1988*, Sydney: National Perinatal Statistics Unit.

Navot, D., Berge, P.A., Williams, M.A., Carrisi, G.J., Guzman, I., Sandler, B. and Grunfeld, L. (1991) 'Poor oocyte quality rather than implantation failure as a cause of age-related decline', *Lancet*, 337, 1375–7.

Navot, D., Relou, A., Birkenfield, A., Rabinowitz, R., Brzezinski, A. and Margalioth, E. J. (1988) 'Risk factors and prognostic variables in the ovarian hyperstimulation syndrome', *American Journal of Obstetrics and Gynaecology*, 159, 210–15.

Needham, J. (1959) A History of Embryology, Cambridge: Cambridge University Press.

New England Journal of Medicine (Editorial) (1937) 'Conception in a watch glass', 217, 678–9.

Okely, J. (1983) *The Traveller-Gypsies*, Cambridge: Cambridge University Press.

Parkin, R. (1997) *Kinship: An Introduction to the Basic Concepts*, London: Blackwell.

Peters, H., Nervell, S.J. and Obhrai, M. (1991) 'Impact of assisted reproduction on neonatal care', *Lancet*, 337, 797.

Pfeffer, N. (1987) 'Artificial insemination, in-vitro fertilisation and the stigma of infertility', in M. Stanworth (ed.), *Reproductive Technologies: Gender, Motherhood and Medicine*, Oxford: Polity Press.

—— (1992) 'From private patients to privatization: a brief history for the treatment of infertility in England and Wales', in M. Stacey (ed.), *Changing Human Reproduction: Social Science Perspectives*, London: Sage.

Piette, C., de Mouzon, J., Bachelot, A. and Spira, A. (1990) 'In vitro fertilisation: influence of women's age on pregnancy rates', *Human Reproduction*, 5, 56–9.

Power, M., Baber, R., Abdalla, H., Kirkland, A., Leonard, T.S. and Studd, J.W. W. (1990) 'A comparison of the attitudes of volunteer donors and infertile patient donors on an ovum donation programme', *Human Reproduction*, 5, 352–5.

Price, F. (1988) 'Establishing guidelines: regulation and the clinical management of infertility', in R. Lee and D. Morgan (eds), *Birthrights: Law and Ethics at the Beginning of Life*, London: Routledge.

—— (1989) *The Parents' Study: Final Report to the Department of Health*, lodged in the Department of Health Library, London.

—— (1990a) 'The management of uncertainty in obstetric practice: ultrasonography, in vitro fertilisation and embryo transfer', in M. McNeil *et al.* (eds), *The New Reproductive Technologies*, London: Macmillan.

—— (1990b) 'Who helps?', in B.J. Botting, A.J. Macfarlane and F.V. Price (eds), *Three, Four and More: A Study of Triplets and Higher Order Births*, London: Her Majesty's Stationery Office.

—— (1990c) 'Consequences', in B.J. Botting, A.J. Macfarlane and F.V. Price (eds), *Three, Four and More: A Study of Triplets and Higher Order Births*, London: Her Majesty's Stationery Office.

—— (1991) 'Isn't she coping well?', in Roberts, H. (ed.), *Women's Health Matters*, London: Routledge.

—— (1992), 'Framing science: women confront expertise in the clinic', paper presented at the Science Policy Support Group 'Women in Science' Forum, London.

—— (1995) 'Conceiving relations: egg and sperm donation in assisted procreation', in D. Pearl and R. Pickford (eds), *Frontiers of Family Law II*, London: John Wiley.

—— (1996) 'Now you see it, now you don't: mediating science and managing uncertainty in reproductive medicine', in A. Irwin, and B. Wynne, (eds), *Misunderstanding Science? The Public Reconstruction of Science and Technology*, Cambridge: Cambridge University Press.

—— (1997) 'Matchmaking in the clinic: gamete donation and the management of difference', in A. Clarke, and E. Parsons, (eds), *Culture, Kinship and Genes: Towards Cross-cultural Genetics*, London: Macmillan.

—— (1998) *Collaborative conceptions: the social implications of egg donation*, End-of-grant report, London: Nuffield Foundation.

Ragoné, Helena (1994) *Surrogate Motherhood: Conception in the Heart*, Boulder, CO: Westview Press.

Rapp, R. (1987) 'Moral pioneers: women, men and fetuses on a frontier of reproductive technology', *Women and Health*, 13(1/2), 101–16.

—— (1995) 'Heredity, or revising the facts of life', in S. J. Yanagisako and C. Delancy (eds), *Naturalizing Power: Essays in Feminist Cultural Analysis*, New York: Routledge.

Ravetz, J. (1990) 'Knowledge in an uncertain world', *New Scientist*, 22 September, 18.

Rivière, P. (1985) 'Unscrambling parenthood: the Warnock Report', *Anthropology Today*, 4, 2–7.

Rock, J. and Menkin, M. (1944) 'In vitro fertilisation and cleavage of human ovarian eggs', *Science*, 100, 105–7.

Saifullah Khan, V. (1977) 'The Pakistanis: Mirpuri villagers at home and in Bradford', in J.L. Watson (ed.), *Between Two Cultures*, Oxford: Basil Blackwell.

Sandelowski, M. (1993) *With Child in Mind: Studies of the Personal Encounter with Infertility*, Philadelphia, PA: University of Pennsylvania Press.

Sauer, M.V. (1996) 'Oocyte donation: reflections on past work and future directions', *Human Reproduction*, 11, 1149–50.

—— (1997) 'Exploitation or woman's right?' *British Medical Journal*, 314, 1403.

Sauer, M.V., Paulson, R.J. and Lobo, R.A. (1990) 'A preliminary report on oocyte donation extending reproductive potential to women over 40', *New England Journal of Medicine*, 323, 1157–60.

Schneider, D.M. (1968) *American Kinship: A Cultural Account*, Englewood Cliffs, N.J: Prentice-Hall.

—— (1980) *American Kinship: A Cultural Account* (2nd Edition), Chicago, IL: University of Chicago Press.

—— (1984) *A Critique of the Study of Kinship*, Ann Arbor, MI: University of Michigan Press.

—— (1992) Comment on 'Virgin births and sterile debates: anthropology and New Reproductive Technologies' by C. Shore, *Current Anthropology*, 33, 307–10.

Schover, L.R., Reis, J., Collins, R.L., Blankstein, J., Kanoti, C. and Quigley, M.M. (1990) 'The psychological evaluation of oocyte donors', *Journal of Psychosomatic Obstetrics and Gynaecology*, 11, 299–309.

Schwartz, D., Mayaux, M. J. and Federation CECOS (1982) 'Female fecundity as a function of age: results of artificial insemination in 2193 multiparous women with azoospermic husbands', *New England Journal of Medicine*, 306, 404–6.

Scott-Jupp, R., Field, D.M. and Macfadyen, U. (1991) 'Multiple pregnancies resulting from assisted conception: burden on neonatal units', *British Medical Journal*, 302, 1079.

Segalen, M. (1986) *Historical Anthropology of the Family* (trans. J.C. Whitehouse and S. Matthews), Cambridge: Cambridge University Press.

Seibel, M. (1988) 'A new era in reproductive technology', *New England Journal of Medicine*, 318, 828–34.

Seppala, M. (1985) 'The world collaborative report of in vitro fertilisation and embryo replacement: current state of the art in 1984', in M. Seppala and R. G. Edwards (eds), 'In Vitro Fertilisation and Embryo Transfer', *Annals of the New York Academy of Science*, 442, 558–63.

Serhal, P. (1990) 'Oocyte donation and surrogacy', in R.G. Edwards (ed.), 'Assisted Human Conception', *British Medical Bulletin*, 46, 796–812.

Serhal, P.F. and Craft, I.L. (1989) 'Oocyte donation in 61 patients', *Lancet*, 1, 1185–7.

Serr, D.M., Tyano, S., Zabner, L. and Levran, D. (1989) 'Psychosocial implications of egg donation', *Ethical Problems in Reproductive Medicine*, 31–3.

Silverstone, R. and Hirsch, E. (eds) (1992) *Consuming Technologies*, London: Routledge.

Smith, B.H. and Cooke, I.D. (1991) 'Ovarian hyperstimulation: actual and theoretical risks', *British Medical Journal*, 302, 127–8.

Snowden, R. (1990) 'The family and artificial reproduction', in D.R. Bromham, M.E. Dalton and J.C. Jackson (eds), *Philosophical Ethics in Reproductive Medicine*, Manchester: Manchester University Press.

Snowden, R. and Mitchell, C.D. (1981) *The Artificial Family: A Consideration of Artificial Insemination by Donor*, London: Unwin.

Snowden, R., Mitchell, C.D. and Snowden, E. (1983) *Artificial Reproduction: A Social Investigation*, London: George Allen and Unwin.

Spallone, P. (1992) *Generation Games: Genetic Engineering and the Future for our Lives*, London: The Women's Press.

—— (1996) 'The Salutary Tale of the Pre-Embryo', in N. Lykke and R. Braidotti, (eds), *Between Monsters, Goddesses and Cyborgs: Feminist Confrontations with Media, Medicine, and Cyberspace*, London: Zed Press.

Spallone, P. and Steinberg, D.L. (eds) (1987) *Made to Order: The Myth of Reproductive and Genetic Progress*, Oxford: Pergamon Press.

Spiro, M. (1968) 'Virgin birth, parthenogenesis and physiological paternity: an essay in cultural interpretation', *Man*, 3, 242–61.

Stacey, M. (ed.) (1992) *Changing Human Reproduction: A Social Science Perspective*, London: Sage.

Stanworth, M. (ed.) (1987) *Reproductive Technologies: Gender, Motherhood and Medicine*, Cambridge: Polity Press.

Stein, Z.A. (1985) 'A woman's age: childbearing and child rearing', *American Journal of Epidemiology*, 121, 327–43.

Steven, C. (1987) 'Test-tube sisters', *Independent*, 29 September, 13.

Stolcke, V. (1986) 'New reproductive technologies – same old fatherhood', *Critique of Anthropology*, 6, 5–32.

—— (1998) 'El Sexo de la bitecnología', in A. Durán and J. Reichman (eds), *Genes en el Laborotorio y en la Fabrica*, Madrid: Editorial Trotta and Fundación Tero de Mayo.

Strathern, M. (1981) *Kinship at the Core: An Anthropology of Elmdon, a Village in North-west Essex in the 1960s*, Cambridge: Cambridge University Press.

—— (1988) *The Gender of the Gift: Problems with Women and Problems with Society in Melanesia*, Berkeley and Los Angeles: California University Press.

—— (1991a) *Partial Connections* A.S.A.O. Special Publication 3, Savage, MD: Rowman and Littlefield.

—— (1991b) 'Partners and consumers: making relations visible', *New Literary History*, 22, 581–601.

—— (1992a) *After Nature: English Kinship in the Late Twentieth Century*, Cambridge: Cambridge University Press.

—— (1992b) *Reproducing the Future: Essays on Anthropology, Kinship and the New Reproductive Technologies*, Manchester: Manchester University Press.

—— (1992c) 'Reproducing Anthropology', in S. Wallman (ed.), *Contemporary Futures*, London: Routledge.

—— (1995) 'The nice thing about culture is that everyone has it', in M. Strathern (ed.), *Shifting contexts: Transformations in Anthroplogical Knowledge*, London: Routledge.

—— (1996) 'Gender: division or comparison?', in N. Charles and F. Hughes-Freeland (eds), *Practising Feminism: Identity, Difference, Power*, London: Routledge.

Thompson, K. (1997) 'Regulation, de-regulation and re-regulation', in K. Thompson (ed.), *Media and Cultural Regulation*, London: Sage.

Trounson, A., Leeton, J., Besanko, M., Wood, C. and Conti, A. (1983) 'Pregnancy established in an infertile patient after transfer of a donated embryo fertilised in vitro', *British Medical Journal*, 286, 835.

Trounson, A.O. and Wood, C. (1984) 'In vitro fertilisation results, 1979–82, at Monash University, Queen Victoria and Epworth Medical Centres', *Journal of In Vitro Fertilisation and Embryo Transfer*, 1, 42–7.

van Noord-Zaadstra, B.M., Looman, C.W.N., Alsbach, H., Habbema, J.D.F., te Velde, E.R. and Karbaat, J. (1991) 'Delayed childbearing: effect of age on fecundity and outcome of pregnancy', *British Journal of Medicine*, 302, 1361–5.

Veitch, A. (1987) 'Three became mothers with eggs from sisters', *Guardian*, 5 April, 3.

Voluntary Licensing Authority (Joint Medical Research Council/Royal College of Obstetrics and Gynaecologists) (1986) *The First Report of the Voluntary Licensing Authority for Human 'In-Vitro' Fertilisation and Embryology*, London: VLA.

—— (1987) *The Second Report of the Voluntary Licensing Authority for Human 'In-Vitro' Fertilisation and Embryology*, London: VLA.

Wagner, R. (1972) *Habu: The Innovation of Meaning in Daribi Religion*, Chicago: University of Chicago Press.

—— (1978) *Lethal Speech: Daribi Myth as Symbolic Obviation*, Ithaca, NY: Cornell University Press.

—— (1986) *Symbols that Stand for Themselves*, Chicago, IL: University of Chicago Press.

Wallman, S. (1984) *Eight London Households*, London: Tavistock.

Warnock, M. (1985) *A Question of Life: The Warnock Report on Human Fertilisation and Embryology*, Oxford: Basil Blackwell.

Waterstone, J., Parsons, J. and Bolton, V. (1991) 'Elective transfer of two embryos', *Lancet*, 337, 975–6.

Weir, L. (1996) 'Recent developments in the government of pregnancy', *Economy and Society*, 25, 372–92.

Weir, L. and Habib, J. (1997) 'A critical feminist analysis of the Final Report of the [Canadian] Royal Commission on New Reproductive Technologies', in *Studies in Political Economy*, 52: 137–54.

Werbner, P. (1990) *The Migration Process: Capital, Gifts and Offerings among British Pakistanis*, Oxford: Berg.

Westmore, A. (1984) 'History', in C. Wood and A. Trounson (eds), *Clinical In Vitro Fertilisation*, Berlin: Springer.

Weston, K. (1991) *Families We Choose: Lesbians, Gays, Kinship*, New York, NY: Columbia University Press.

Whiteford, L. M. and Poland, M. L. (1989) *New Approaches to Human Reproduction: Social and Ethical Dimensions*, Boulder, CO: Westview Press.

Wilmut, I., Schnieke A.K., McWhir, J., Kind, A.J. and Campbell, K.H.S. (1997)

'Viable offspring derived from fetal and adult mammalian cells', *Nature*, 385: 810–13.

Winston, R.M.L. (1991) 'Resources for infertility treatment', in W.A.W. Walters (ed.), 'Human reproduction: current and future ethical issues', *Baillière's Clinical Obstetrics and Gynaecology*, 5, 551–73.

—— (1997) 'The promise of cloning for human medicine', *British Medical Journal*, 314, 913–14.

Wolfram, S. (1987) *In Laws and Outlaws: Kinship and Marriage in England*, London: Croom Helm.

—— (1989) 'Surrogacy in the United Kingdom', in L.M. Whiteford and M.L. Poland (eds), *New Approaches to Human Reproduction: Social and Ethical Dimensions*, London: Westview Press.

Wynne, B. (1991) 'Public perception and communication of risk: what do we know?' *Journal of National Institutes of Health Research*, 3, 65–70.

Yoxen, E. (1988) 'Public concern and the steering of science', Report for the Science Policy Support Group, Nottingham.

—— (1990) 'Conflicting concerns: the political context of recent embryo research policy in Britain', in M. McNeil *et al.* (eds), *The New Reproductive Technologies*, London: Macmillan.

Index